What's *with* Fiber?

GENE & MONICA SPILLER

D1571385

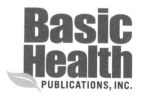

Basic Health
PUBLICATIONS, INC.

The information contained in this book is based upon the research and personal and professional experiences of the authors. It is not intended as a substitute for consulting with your physician or other healthcare provider. Any attempt to diagnose and treat an illness should be done under the direction of a healthcare professional.

The publisher does not advocate the use of any particular healthcare protocol but believes the information in this book should be available to the public. The publisher and authors are not responsible for any adverse effects or consequences resulting from the use of the suggestions, preparations, or procedures discussed in this book. Should the reader have any questions concerning the appropriateness of any procedures or preparation mentioned, the authors and the publisher strongly suggest consulting a professional healthcare advisor.

Basic Health Publications, Inc.
28812 Top of the World Drive
Laguna Beach, CA 92651
800-575-8890

Library of Congress Cataloging-in-Publication Data

Spiller, Gene A.
    What's with fiber? : enjoy better health with a high-fiber, plant-based diet / Gene and Monica Spiller.
        p. cm.
    Includes bibliographical references and index.
    ISBN-13: 978-1-59120-111-3
    ISBN-10: 1-59120-111-X
  1. High-fiber diet. 2. Fiber in human nutrition. I. Spiller, Monica II. Title.

    RM237.6.S65   2005
    613.2'63—dc22

                                                            2005015024

Editor: Roberta W. Waddell
Typesetting/Book design: Gary A. Rosenberg
Cover design: Mike Stromberg

Printed in the United States of America

10   9   8   7   6   5   4   3   2   1

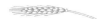

Contents

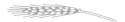

*This book is dedicated to the pioneers of fiber in nutrition and health,
Captain Surgeon T. L. Cleave and Dr. Alexander Walker,
and to Drs. Hugh Trowell and Denis Burkitt who discovered them.
They all inspired us far beyond the scientific concepts they promoted,
opening a new era in nutrition and disease prevention.
We are also dedicating it to all the people of the world who
find better health in a high-fiber, plant-based diet.*

Acknowledgments

This book would not have been possible without our frequent interactions over more than thirty years with many researchers and writers in the fields of nutrition and fiber. And thanks to our discussions over the past twenty years with many of the authors of scientific chapters in the *CRC Handbook of Fiber in Human Nutrition,* we have developed a unique insight into what fiber and phytonutrients can do. We would especially like to thank the three physician-researchers James Anderson, Antonia Tricholoupou, and David Jenkins, who gave us their personal viewpoints, included in this book.

Alexa and Marika Bruce have helped search and condense the research work that goes back to the 1970s and continues now. Rosemary Schmele and Ann Gunderson have given us valuable suggestions on selected parts of the text. Antonella Dewell helped with preparation of the charts and tables in the appendices. John Richards of Menlo Park, California, has created the drawings that illustrate, in a simple way, the magic of a plant.

We thank our publisher, Norman Goldfind, for his decision to publish this book, and our thanks also to Roberta Waddell who edited it.

Introduction

What's with fiber? All our plant food is built with fiber and is ours for the eating, provided we eat plant foods whole. This book presents the fascinating history of fiber, its consumption patterns through the ages, and the evolution of refined foods for the rich and unrefined foods for the poor. You will read how the tremendous diversity of fibers helps to ensure that all types of fiber are present in the diet. People are told to eat at least 25 grams of fiber each day, but not told of the need for a variety of fiber, or that 25 grams should be the *minimum* intake, far from the ideal 30–50 grams daily. This valuable, but often overlooked, information will be stressed throughout the book.

What's with Fiber emphasizes that, in order to obtain enough fiber and phytonutrients (plant nutrients), you need to eat a plant-based diet that is naturally high in fiber. High-fiber foods and their nutrient-rich extracts will help you achieve better health and prevent disease, while enjoying great whole, natural foods.

Is fiber a magic healer and disease-prevention wonder? Are fibers from different foods the same or different? And what about all the nutrients and the newly discovered phytochemicals—many of them highly protective and beneficial—that exist with fiber in food? What the many different kinds of fiber all have in common is that, except for a tiny amount of animal foods, such as the edible shells in softshell crabs, they are found only in plants.

Recent headlines talk about overweight and obesity becoming one of the major causes of death in the United States, surpassing cigarette smoking. The last hundred years have seen a decline in death from infectious diseases and an increase in deaths from degenerative diseases, such as cancer, diabetes, and heart disease.

There is no doubt that, with obesity currently epidemic in the Western world, increasing the consumption of fiber-containing foods and decreasing the intake of refined foods—refined grains and fiber-free animal products, such as meats—will help prevent overweight and obesity and their sad health consequences.

The press continually reminds people of the health problems that are prevalent in this millennium, and the chronic diseases that are related to Western lifestyles, almost all of which are related to low-fiber, refined-food diets. "World Facing Diabetes Catastrophe" was the headline of a recent Reuters news item about a conference on diabetes in Paris. Dr. James Anderson, who has studied diabetes and fiber for decades, says, "Diabetes mellitus is emerging as a major health problem throughout the world, and current evidence suggests that increased fat intake and decreased fiber intake may contribute." Although diabetes is linked to a higher risk for heart disease and other health problems, it does not have to be a catastrophe. This runaway disease can be effectively reduced simply by combining a high-fiber, whole-plant-food diet with reasonable physical activity.

In this book, we answer key questions about the relationship of fiber and its protective compounds to health. We present the science behind fiber and phytochemicals, and we include all the fibers found in different foods and the nutrients and phytochemicals that come with fiber. In this highly accessible, easy-to-read book, we remind you of the important point that, as with refined flours for example, many nutrients are lost when the fiber is removed in the process of refining plant foods, such as grains. Although some nutrients may remain after the fiber is removed, as in fresh fruit and vegetable juices, and such ancient beverages as green tea, these super sources of many precious nutrients should be used only as *additions* to a high-fiber diet, *not in place of* whole fruits and vegetables.

We discuss how the birth of the phytochemical-antioxidant era in the 1990s confirms that *reductionist* research (which desperately tries to attribute the development of a disease to a lack of *just one* food component, such as fiber) can lead to conflicting results. We remind you that there is more to fiber than celery strings or wheat bran. And we do it using very little medical jargon. The book is designed to give you a user-friendly, readable overview of the benefits of individual plant foods.

Part One helps you understand what fiber is and what comes with it in natural unrefined plant foods. Part Two explores the fascinating history of fiber, going back thousands of years, and coming up to the era that started in the 1970s when the researchers T. L. Cleave, Alexander Walker, Hugh Trowell, and Denis Burkitt opened the door to the current fiber era. We present the history as well as the practical side of fiber in the diet because we believe it can help people understand the inner workings of better health. We define *reductionism* and its pros and cons, and we define the various types of fiber and phytochemicals, from antioxidants to tartaric acid. We discuss in depth the relation of fiber, and what goes with it, to good health and the prevention of many chronic diseases—from cancer to diabetes and heart disease. We take a look at the health of some primitive populations and show what happens when these people move into cities and change to more refined diets.

Part Three explores beans, lentils, nuts, peas, and whole grains; the flowers, leaves, roots, and stems we call vegetables; vegetation from the sea; fungi; and fresh and dried fruits of all colors and shapes. Finding out what is present in all these plant foods will give you a better understanding of their health-giving wonders. In Part Three, we also discuss extracts of high-fiber foods, such as teas, and fruit and vegetable juices, and their place in a food plan.

There are Appendices in the back, which have tables and graphs with data on fiber, and these are followed by a Glossary and sections containing Resources and References. An Index completes the book.

Remembering
a Key Encounter

It was January 1977 in Palo Alto, California, a small city just south of San Francisco. The sun was warm and the grass was already green on the hills following the fall rains. The yellow flowers of the wild mustard gave the hills the touch of spring that is typical of the San Francisco Bay area, a region that never sees a true winter.

As I drove to the San Francisco airport, I sensed that the two people I was about to bring back to Palo Alto with me—Drs. Denis Burkitt and Hugh Trowell from England—would have a deep influence on the rest of my life. These two physicians, whom I like to call the fathers of modern fiber in nutrition, were coming to Palo Alto to give a major presentation to our nutrition research group at Syntex Research. I had briefly met them before and had had some correspondence with them. I had written about them in medical books and scientific reviews on food fibers, and had talked on the phone with them to arrange this meeting. I had also had a brief meeting with Dr. Burkitt at a fiber conference in Canada in 1976. But now we would have a chance to spend a few days together in both formal and informal meetings, the latter often leading to a freer, more productive and creative exchange of ideas.

During these meetings with Drs. Burkitt and Trowell, we established a major connection, one that deepened throughout the remainder of their lives (Dr. Trowell passed away in the late 1980s and Dr. Burkitt, in the early '90s). We still feel the influence of their ideas on our own research.

The study of dietary fiber has come a long way since then. When I edited my first scientific book on fiber in 1975, *Fiber in Human Nutrition,* I had a difficult time finding enough medical experts and scientists to write chapters for the book. Yet only a few years later, in 1982, when I edited the first edition of the *CRC Handbook of Dietary Fiber in Human Nutrition,* the work of Drs.

Burkitt and Trowell had ignited so many fires in the minds of people in the medical community that I not only had no problem finding enough authors for that book, I had the difficult task of leaving many researchers' contributions out of the book for lack of space.

—Gene Spiller

PART ONE

What Is Fiber and What Comes with It?

1

What Is Fiber?

The Walls of the Plant Cell

Picture a plant cell in a fruit, leaf, root, seed, or stem. It is fiber that gives the structure to the walls of these cells that hold the fluids, including water, and all the nutrients and other vital components inside the cell. There may be some gum and mucilage (also classified as fiber) inside the cell—the gummy substances in okra, for example—but the principal amount of fiber eaten is from the wall of the cell.

Fiber can look like a celery string. It's what's left behind when you make apple, carrot, or orange juice. Sadly, fiber is also what's mostly left behind when you sift wholegrain flour to make refined white flour.

In discussing health and disease, it is important to define fiber as that part of fruits, grains, nuts, seeds, and vegetables that is not broken down by the enzymes in your digestive system, and so is not absorbed the way you absorb fats, proteins, and carbohydrate (starch and sugars). The fact that fiber is not digested by the enzymes in the stomach and small intestine previously led many to consider fiber a worthless component to be discarded (as in bran from wheat, or rice polishings from rice).

Instead, fiber is not digested until it reaches the lactic bacteria *in the large intestine* at the end of the digestive system. This is the colon where microorganisms live that can break down the most soluble fiber and *digest* it, producing vinegar acid (acetic acid) and other similar short-chain fatty acids. These acids are beneficial to the health of the colon and are absorbed by it to supply some calories.

Insoluble fibers are not digested at all, even by the bacteria, but give bulk to the stool and keep it moist and easy to eliminate. An adequate intake of insoluble fiber prevents and relieves constipation.

Fiber Is Mostly Carbohydrate

Plants are built from carbohydrates. They are, after all, the most common material produced by green leaves in sunlight during photosynthesis, from water and the carbon dioxide in the air. These carbohydrates range from the smallest sugars to huge polymers, or chains, of these small sugar units.

Glucose and *fructose* are familiar *simple sugars* that plants make. So also is *sucrose,* which is built from just two sugar units, or molecules—one each of fructose and glucose. Simple sugars dissolve easily in water, taste very sweet, and are easily digested.

These sugars can link up to make polymers, or chains and branched chains, of varying lengths. The longer and stronger the polymers, the less they will be able to dissolve in water, taste sweet, or be digested.

Starch is a medium-strong polymer of glucose (not sweet-tasting) that forms a gel in water, and can still be digested in the stomach. Other sugar polymers, such as *inulin,* also make gels in water that sometimes taste very sweet, yet cannot be broken down by digestive enzymes to be digested in the stomach. Unlike starch, the sweet-tasting inulin is a *soluble dietary fiber* because it is not digested until it reaches the bacteria of the colon.

The longest and strongest sugar polymers, such as *cellulose,* an *insoluble dietary fiber,* do not dissolve in water. Although they do absorb and hold water like a sponge, they cannot be digested, even by the bacteria in the colon.

In summary, plant carbohydrates can be classified as:

- Energy foods that are completely digested (glucose, cane sugar, starch);

- Soluble fiber that is not digested until it reaches the bacteria in the colon (*see* Table 1.1);

- Insoluble fiber that is not digested at all and serves as bulk (*see* Table 1.2).

TABLE 1.1 SOLUBLE FIBERS	
Soluble Fiber	Source
Beta-glucan	Oats, barley
Inulin or fructo-oligosaccharide (FOS)	Chicory, Jerusalem artichokes
Pectin	Apples, beets, orange peel
Pentosans	Rye, wheat

TABLE 1.2 INSOLUBLE FIBERS	
Insoluble Fiber	Source
Agar	Seaweed
Cellulose	Grain and seed brans
Lignin	Grain bran, flaxseed, pears

Quasi-Carbohydrate Fiber

Quasi-carbohydrate fiber is a made-up term to describe foodstuffs that fall outside the description of a carbohydrate, but resemble carbohydrate fiber because they remain undigested until they reach the colon. *Tartaric acid,* richly present in grapes, and *sorbitol,* found in cherries, are examples. Both compounds remain undigested until they reach the colonic bacteria.

Resistant-Starch Fiber

Cooking and processing plant foods can have the effect of changing digestible energy food into indigestible fiber. This commonly happens to a small amount of the starch in wheat when it is made into pasta or bread. The starch is changed into a form that resists digestion until it reaches the bacteria of the colon. It is therefore classified as soluble fiber. Hans Englyst in England was the first to give it the name resistant starch. It is not usually listed on food labels, but appears as part of the dietary fiber content.

Soluble Fiber Provides Few Calories and a Good Cholesterol Profile

How does soluble fiber contribute calories and moderate the metabolic processes in the human body? When soluble fiber reaches the colon and is digested, or fermented, by the microorganisms in the colon, certain short-chain fatty acids are produced, such as acetic acid (found in vinegar), butyric acid (found in butter), and propionic acid (found in cheese). These short-chain fatty acids are absorbed into the blood, and provide energy calories.

There are three major advantages to this process. First, these acids supply only half the calories that would be expected based on the original carbohydrate content of the soluble fiber. Soluble fiber and resistant starch contribute 2 calories per gram, due to the metabolism of the short-chain fatty acids, while digestible carbohydrates supply 4 calories per gram. Secondly, the effect of these short-chain fatty acids is to improve the cholesterol profile in your blood; they favor the high-density lipoproteins, the HDL (good) cholesterol. A third advantageous effect of soluble fiber is that it promotes the growth of lactic bacteria that can add bulk in the colon and improve immunity to infections.

Insoluble Fiber

The task for insoluble fiber in the body is to carry water and food through the entire digestive system. By the time a meal reaches the colon, the digestible food has been absorbed. Then, as it enters the colon, the soluble fiber becomes digested by the bacteria. Finally, the insoluble fiber carries the bacteria and undigested excess food and bile through the colon for elimination as stools. Insoluble fiber absorbs water, swells like a sponge, and keeps the colon properly filled and able to promote easy elimination.

Insoluble fiber, in the form of cellulose, is found in large amounts only in the bran coats of grains. Beans and lentils are moderately rich in cellulose, but in fruits and vegetables, the cellulose is greatly diluted by the high water content. This means that eating sufficient quantities of whole grains, and therefore grain bran, is the only way to ensure a healthful intake of insoluble fiber.

Lignin is in the woody cells of plants, and is present only in very small amounts in some plant foods. It is also classified as insoluble dietary fiber because it resists digestion even by the bacteria of the colon, but it is not a carbohydrate in the scientific sense, but is instead a large polymer of phenolic compounds.

How Much Fiber Do You Need?

You need between 25 and 50 grams a day according to your height. Children need fiber too and should be eating grains in the wholegrain form, and plenty of fruits and vegetables, from the time they are weaned. In general, if you eat a varied whole-plant-based diet, you will automatically be eating dietary fiber in the right quantity, with the right mix of soluble and insoluble fiber.

Ideally, transit time for your food through your body should be no more than one to two days. The right amount and mix of fiber in the diet will make elimination easy, followed by a feeling of well-being and a flatter abdomen.

Nutrition Labels and Fiber

Nutrition labels on commercially packaged foods often need some interpretation to understand how much of the total carbohydrate is completely digestible (4 calories per gram), how much is soluble fiber (2 calories per gram), and how much is insoluble fiber (0 calories per gram). The amount is usually given for the total carbohydrates in the food, followed by a list of the contributing carbohydrates: dietary fiber, starch, and sugar. Often, one or more of the contributing carbohydrates are missing from the list, and you are left to calculate these yourself by the difference.

What about lignin? Even when present, the contribution of lignin to insoluble fiber is very small, so including all the dietary fiber under the carbohydrate label is a reasonable approximation.

It is also useful to know that protein contributes 4 calories per gram, and fat contributes 9 calories per gram.

If the dietary fiber contribution is missing from the nutrition facts label, or is very small, the product is probably not a whole-plant food. To determine this, compare it with a known whole-plant food version of the product, if possible.

2

Nutrients and Phytochemicals That Come with Fiber

Hundreds of nutrients and phytochemicals come with fiber, and they all play a role in protecting your health. These protective nutrients are missing from refined sugar, refined flours, and white rice. Some progress has been made; for example, white breads now come enriched with some vitamins and minerals. These are good beginning steps, but they are far from being all of the completely beneficial protective compounds found in whole, unrefined foods.

Nutrients Associated with Dietary Fiber

Dietary fiber, often in the form of cellulose and pectin, is the material in the cell walls of plants, which encloses the cell's contents: sugars, starches, proteins, oils, vitamins, minerals, enzymes, and many yet-unknown phytochemicals. But when the cells are compressed, these cell contents can instead be closely associated with the cell walls, which means that they are constituents of the fibrous part of food. This is especially true of grains, which have very little cell-wall material associated with the starch and protein of the endosperm center, but have almost all the other nutrients concentrated in the cells of the outer bran and germ. When the bran and germ are removed from wheat and similar grains, all the vital nutrients, such as vitamins B and E, and minerals, are also removed. The classic case always cited in the history of nutrition is the discovery in Southeast Asia that making brown rice white by removing the outside fibrous layer of bran and germ caused a deficiency of vitamin B_1 (thiamine), which resulted in beriberi disease. This revelation was the beginning of the science of vitamins, and the list goes on from there.

People's digestive systems work best when whole-plant foods are the source for ingesting sugars, starch, protein, and oils, and they should be the foundation of the diet.

Phytonutrients with Fiber

In the past, relatively few plants were considered capable of supplying medicinal and biologically active compounds. To accommodate the long list of interesting compounds now discovered to exist in all plants, including food plants, the terms phytonutrients and phytochemicals (phyto = plant) are being used. Some of these phytochemicals, such as phytic acid and tannins, were once seen as *anti*-nutrients to be avoided, but research has shown that these, in particular, are useful in the diet in order to remain in good health.

Phytic acid, which was generally seen only as a binder of minerals, is now recognized as an anti-cancer compound (*see* Chapter 10). And tannins (polyphenolics), once seen as inhibitors of weight gain in animals, are now seen, not only as protectors of the plants in which they naturally occur, but also as antioxidant protectors against many chronic diseases, such as cancer, cardiovascular disease, and diabetes.

The Saas Fee Swiss Declaration

In 1992, a group of international preventive-medicine researchers in the fields of antioxidants and free radicals—those damaging byproducts of energy production in our bodies—held a meeting in Saas Fee, Switzerland and issued a declaration, afterward signed by all present and later by hundreds of researchers worldwide.

One researcher, Lester Packer, said of the encouraging findings of the previous fifteen years: "Compelling evidence indicates that multiple servings of fruits and vegetables in the daily diet provide health benefits. Similarly, health benefits of beverages, such as tea and red wine, have been reported. The phytonutrients suspected to be involved are polyphenolics. These and other phytonutrients may also account for the beneficial effects of plant extracts from gingko leaves and pine bark, which have been used as traditional herbal medicines for centuries."

Whole-Plant Foods—The Foundation of Life

Plants make their own necessary compounds by using very simple materials, such as water and minerals from the soil, and by making use of carbon dioxide from the air and energy from the sun to synthesize vital compounds. Not so, for animals and humans who depend on food plants and their many wonderful compounds to maintain life. Whether people eat an all-plant vegan diet, or an omnivorous diet that includes meats and dairy products, everyone is nevertheless totally dependent on plants for food. Within the plant cells is an enormous capacity to make and store compounds that can only be ingested by eating plant foods, or flesh from animals that have eaten plant foods, or have eaten other animals that have eaten plant foods. This is the food chain. Eating low on the food chain means eating plant foods as the foundation of the diet, and eating high on the food chain means making animal products the foundation of the diet. Either way, plants are the essential ingredient.

The beneficial effects of whole-plant foods are not yet fully understood, and often go beyond the benefits that can be predicted from the separate compounds found in plants. Whole grains are a good example. Many times, wholegrain foods give valuable protection against cancer, cardiovascular disease, diabetes, and obesity, but this protection often diminishes when only isolated parts of the grains are eaten.

The Magic of Polyphenols

Polyphenols (also known as polyphenolics) are closely associated with the fiber in the walls of cells. There are hundreds of different polyphenolics in plants, but they all have an ability to protect the plant from too much oxygen and ultraviolet (UV) light. They are often beautifully colored, and they have various healthful effects as part of the diet. Sometimes the polyphenolics in the cell walls are woody lignins, which are not digested by enzymes and are therefore insoluble dietary fiber. Smaller polyphenolic units known as lignans can also be present and these can be released during digestion and absorbed. Some lignans are *phytoestrogens* (plant estrogens), and also antioxidants, and this combination makes them protective against breast cancer. In plant foods, lignins and lignans are most frequently associated with the cell-wall fiber in seed coats, the outside layer, of seeds—as in flax and grain seeds, for example.

The plant cells on the outside of the plant usually contain high concentrations of polyphenolics, and many of these are easily absorbed in the intestines. The rich colors in the skins of fruit are usually antioxidant polyphenolics. They have medicinal properties, they help to fight inflammation and reduce the fragility of the capillaries. They reduce the effects of diabetes by protecting the capillaries, and also help protect against edema, the accumulation of fluids in the body that can lead to swollen legs or other swelling problems. They can protect against UV radiation, allowing sun on the skin with less damage. Many of these brilliantly colored polyphenolics are easily absorbed because they are water soluble and can enter the cells of the body with great speed. Studies in our center to test how fast antioxidants enter the body show that antioxidant polyphenolics enter the blood approximately fifteen to sixty minutes after being ingested. They do not stay there for long. Soon they leave the blood to enter various organs and cells inside the body.

The well-known French paradox—the fact that the French eat gourmet food, quite high in fat, yet have much lower rates of cardiovascular disease than people in the United States—is usually explained by the red wine that French people drink. Researchers consider the high concentration of red polyphenols in wine one of the reasons for its benefits, but don't forget that the French also eat plenty of fruits and vegetables, which supply even more antioxidant polyphenols.

The Not-So-Colorful Polyphenols

There is another group of brown antioxidant polyphenolics, known as tannins, that are found, often with lignans, in high concentrations in the cells of seed coats, especially in the bran of grains. Although other antioxidants, such as vitamin E, are also present in whole grains, the whole-grain polyphenolics make a very important contribution to fighting cardiovascular disease and preventing diabetes. Whole grains contribute polyphenols just as vitally as fruits and vegetables in the diet—a serving of whole grains can provide as much antioxidant activity as a serving of fruit, and more than a serving of most vegetables.

Other polyphenols are colorless, and they are recognizable by their tendency to rapidly become brown. A cut apple or artichoke turns brown at the site of a cut or injury by an insect because the polyphenolics become oxidized and the color of the oxidized polyphenolic is brown, at least on the surface. You can prevent this discoloration by coating the cut surface with another antioxidant, such as vitamin C. Lemon juice, high in antioxidant vitamin C, is perfect for this.

Is It the Fiber, the Polyphenols, or Both That Have an Effect?

In the early 1990s, researchers at last began to appreciate the contribution that polyphenols made to people's well-being. The main effect, due to soluble fiber alone, seems to be that it is fermentable by the bacteria in the colon. Short-chain fatty acids that can be absorbed are produced, providing a good cholesterol profile. Insoluble fiber absorbs water and is a bulking agent in the colon.

The conflicting results obtained from studies on the effects of fiber as a protector against cancer, cardiovascular problems, and diabetes can often be explained now by considering the polyphenolics. The fiber in whole food is generally associated with polyphenolics and other phytochemicals. When fiber is purified and tested in studies, the amount of polyphenols remaining varies according to the purification process, giving different results. In an experiment done before the many varieties of fiber and associated compounds were appreciated, purified wood pulp, which is not representative of fiber in whole plants, was added to white bread as a source of dietary fiber. The obvious result of this flawed experiment was that purified wood pulp, which is insoluble fiber, provided none of the phytonutrients that would have been provided by the bran and germ in whole-wheat bread.

Antioxidant Vitamins

When you eat whole foods, the antioxidants found inside the cell—beta-carotene that the body can convert to vitamin A when needed, or vitamins C and E—all work together with the antioxidant polyphenolics. The antioxidant vitamins A, C, and E were given credit for health-giving activity decades before the polyphenolic antioxidants were found to be protective.

In oranges and lemons, vitamin C is protected from oxygen damage by antioxidant polyphenols known as bioflavonoids. Albert Szent-Györgi discovered this in the 1930s, and that is why you find some supplements combining vitamin C with bioflavonoids. Vitamin C, in turn, protects vitamin E.

All the antioxidant compounds work together to protect the plant, and in a similar way they all work in concert to protect people.

Plants provide vitamins A (as beta-carotene), C, and E, which people must get from their diet because the body cannot make them. Other plant compounds known to be part of antioxidant and other key functions in the body's cells include glutathione, lipoic acid, the tocopherols, the tocotrienols, and ubiquinone (coenzyme Q10), to mention a few. The mineral selenium is part of this concert of antioxidants, and it too is supplied by plants. Whole plant cells can, in fact, probably supply all the antioxidant compounds needed, both known and as yet unknown.

Waxes and Sterols

Waxes and sterols, both waxy substances, accumulate outside the fiber wall of the cell to protect the fruit, leaves, and other parts of the plant. Plant sterols are similar to cholesterol—a sterol produced by humans and animals—and they can lower blood cholesterol. Before cholesterol-lowering statin drugs took over the market, people with high blood cholesterol used products made with plant sterols to lower their cholesterol, and these are again being pressed into service as replacements for the statins, which can have harmful side effects.

Saponins

Saponins are associated with the fiber in the plant's cell. They are present in many plant foods (perhaps the highest plant source is spinach). They are steroid-like and biologically active to the point of being distinctly poisonous when isolated and concentrated, but washing usually reduces them enough in beans, grains, and vegetables to make them beneficial rather than toxic. Saponins remaining in such plant foods as beans and quinoa will combine with bile acids and cholesterol and cause these to be excreted in the stools, which helps to lower blood cholesterol.

Phytates

All seeds contain phytate (inositol hexaphosphate), sometimes referred to as phytic acid. Seeds also contain a matching enzyme (phytase) that will break it down into inositol and phosphate units when the seed begins to sprout. Phytate is found in the highest amounts in seed foods (beans, flax, grains, and sesame seeds, for example, that could be used to grow new plants). There is relatively little phytate in leafy greens and other vegetables that have no seeds or sprouts.

In grains, the phytate is in the germ and bran. Therefore, refined white flour made only from the wheat endosperm (*see* Chapter 17, Figure 17.2) contains very little phytate, while whole-wheat flour contains practically all the phytate of the grain. The distribution is quite different in beans, lentils, peas, or other legumes where the phytate, in close association with the cell-wall fiber, is distributed throughout the two halves (cotyledens) of the legume.

In seed food, fiber and phytates are so closely associated that fiber's ability to chelate (bind) metal ions is attributed to the presence of the phytates. Fiber itself, especially pectin, can bind with metals, but not as effectively as pure phytates, which can bind with such metal ions as calcium, and zinc. Phytates can also bind with proteins, including digestive enzymes—the starch-digesting enzyme alpha-amylase and the protein-digesting enzyme trypsin, for example. Binding with proteins may be one reason why phytates, together with fiber, produce fewer calories than expected from a food, in comparison with a corresponding amount of refined proteins and starch. The reason many whole-plant foods do not cause the weight gain that refined plant-food fractions do is partly due to the phytates present in the whole, unrefined foods. Other reasons that whole-plant foods are less likely to cause weight gain include the presence of polyphenols and saponins that can also bind with protein.

The role of phytates in the diet that has caused concern in the past has been their ability to bind with metals and cause a deficiency, particularly of zinc. Although zinc deficiencies are rare in diets with an abundant variety of plant and animal foods, deficiencies have arisen in diets limited to processed grains and legumes. In whole-wheat breads, the mineral-binding effects of phytates are reduced in the presence of sprouted grain containing phytase, yeast containing phytase, or lactic bacteria in a sourdough starter that produces acids. But if whole-wheat breads are leavened with baking powder or baking soda, which are alkaline, then minerals such as zinc will bind with phytate. In a diet consisting almost entirely of such bread, this could be a cause of zinc deficiency.

Phytates Are Anti-Cancer

Phytates may also play a role in reducing the incidence of colon cancer. The mechanism for this is not yet clear, but it is believed they bind any excessive iron that could cause damaging oxidation in the colon.

When properly made, both whole-wheat bread and tempeh are regarded as nutritionally superior forms of whole wheat and whole soybeans. A sufficient amount of these foods in a mixed diet can prevent any phytate-induced zinc deficiency and still provide enough remaining phytate for protection against cancer.

B Vitamins and Minerals in Whole-Plant Foods

Many essential nutrients—notably the B vitamins biotin, folic acid, niacin, pantothenic acid, riboflavin, and thiamine—are lost when the grain fiber is removed by sifting wholegrain flour or polishing rice. The B vitamins biotin, niacin, pantothenic acid, riboflavin, and thiamine are necessary for the release of energy from digestible carbohydrates. Folate, vitamin B_6 (pyridoxine), and vitamin B_{12} (cyanocobalamin) are required for the production of new genetic material in order for both plant and animal cells to reproduce.

Whole plant foods can supply all the B vitamins, except B_{12}. And even B_{12} is found in some plant sources, such as seaweeds and mushrooms. However, it should be noted that scientists are not confident that it can be as effectively absorbed as the B_{12} from animal sources, such as meat and eggs.

Many minerals are inside plant cells surrounded by a fiber wall, which serves to underline the crucial role of plant foods in the diet. Plants are an excellent source for relatively large amounts of potassium compared to sodium, and this substance is extremely beneficial for controlling blood pressure. Calcium is sometimes present in quantity in seed cells, such as almonds and sesame. Chlorine, in the form of chloride, is in plant cells, but in insufficient amounts for the stomach to produce enough hydrochloric acid to properly digest food. Sprinkling salt (sodium chloride) on grains or vegetables is a way to compensate for this. Magnesium, seen in its greatest amounts in leafy green vegetables, is present as part of green chlorophyll. Phosphorus is present mostly as phosphate and often as part of phytate.

Trace minerals, such as iron, copper, and zinc, are needed by both plants and animals, but only in small amounts. Other minerals, such as boron, manganese, and selenium, are needed in even smaller amounts by plants, and are more or less present depending on the quantity available from the soil.

Vitamin K

Vitamin K is necessary for healthy blood clotting to prevent uncontrolled blood loss after an injury. Healthy bones are also dependent on vitamin K, which needs daily replenishing. Although animal foods (eggs, meat, and milk) can supply a form of vitamin K, leafy green vegetables, such as chard or kale, eaten daily are a very good source because vitamin K in plants is naturally associated with the fiber of green leaves.

Optimum Diet
for Optimum Health

After reading this chapter, you can understand how rich in nutrients whole, unrefined plant foods are, and why you need to make plant foods a major component of your diet if you desire optimum health. Take a good look at fiber and all that comes with it, and choose a wide variety of whole-plant foods—beans, fruits, nuts and other seeds, vegetables, and whole grains—for an ideal diet.

3

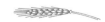

Soluble Fiber
Is Fermented

The Bacteria That Protect

People have been scared of bacteria ever since the 1860s, when Joseph Lister taught everyone to kill bad bacteria that cause infection. Louis Pasteur's message was similar: Kill the bad bacteria in grape juice before you make it into wine. But *good* bacteria are key parts of a healthy digestive system and of many foods that are considered healthy. Cheese, miso (an Asian fermented bean product used to make great soups and sauces), sauerkraut, sourdough breads, wine and beer, and yogurt are all made using good bacteria.

As is common knowledge now, good bacteria are highly concentrated in your colon, and much benefit comes from those that can degrade soluble fiber. The bacterial breakdown of soluble fiber produces short-chain fatty acids, and releases phytonutrients from the plant cells that reach the colon. These released short-chain fatty acids and phytonutrients can be absorbed into the blood from the colon. It should be mentioned that smaller amounts of these beneficial bacteria are also found in the small intestine, which is the twenty-foot digesting and absorbing tube that exits the stomach, and precedes the colon. The small intestine is called *small* because it has a diameter of about one inch, which is much narrower than the large intestine, or colon, with a diameter of about two inches. A significant amount of bacterial breakdown occurs in the small intestine, but most of it happens in the colon.

Some of the most important nutrients that are absorbed after bacterial degradation are the phenolics, which are very protective. They are antioxidant, they protect the capillary blood vessels and the cardiovascular system, and they are anti-cancer and anti-diabetic. Without these good bacteria in the colon, beneficial amounts of phenolic compounds and other phytonutrients would not be available for absorption into the blood. Often the polyphenolics, which are chains of phenolic molecules, cannot be absorbed because they are too large or they are tightly bound to the fiber and would not be released unless the binding fiber was attacked by the good bacteria.

Soluble Fermentable Fiber

Soluble fiber such as gums, pectin, and some hemicelluloses are easily degraded by the bacteria of the colon, leaving the associated cellulose (insoluble fiber) to pass through almost unaffected. As with pectin, various other plant materials remain undigested until they reach the bacteria of the colon. The mucilage from flax seeds, tartaric acid from grapes and grape products, such as raisins, beta-glucans from oats, and seaweed fiber are examples of plant material that is not digested until it reaches the bacteria of the colon. The end products of pectin fermentation by the colonic bacteria are the familiar short-chained fatty acids with small enough molecules to be easily absorbed, such as the acetic acid found in vinegar, the propionic acid often found in cheeses and used as a natural food preservative, and the butyric acid present in butter fat, from which it derives its name. As previously stated, far fewer calories are contributed by pectin and other soluble fiber than by refined sugars and starch, which are completely digested and absorbed. The short-chain acids that are produced as end products of pectin fermentation enter the blood from the colon and supply only half the calories of the original pectin.

When a whole-plant food is eaten, or when the starch has been cooked into a crust, as in breads, some starch can reach the colon before being digested. This is known as resistant starch and it is only broken down by the bacteria once it arrives in the colon. Resistant starch is soluble fiber, and like pectin and other soluble fiber—the bacteria use it for their own energy supply and the body derives the rest of the energy that is available from the absorbed short-chain fatty acids made by the bacteria.

It is possible for simple sugars to reach the colon without having been digested. Chunks of fruit and vegetables are the usual carriers, as well as the various phytonutrients, such as polyphenolics and phytates, that can bind simple sugars. When the fruit or vegetable is broken down by the bacteria in the colon, the sugar is released for use by these bacteria.

Bacteria for a Healthy Colon

A healthy colon is one with a plentiful supply of good bacteria. The healthiest bacteria in the colon are the lactobacillus and the bifidobacteria, which can be as much as 25 percent of all the bacteria present. Bifidobacteria are given the most credit for producing acetic and lactic acids that result in a favorable acidity and a natural inhibition of unfavorable bacteria. There are about four hundred species of bacteria found in the colon, so there is definitely a wealth of detail, much of it yet to be understood. Yeasts are also present in the colon, but in very small numbers compared with the bacteria. Since bacteria are constantly eliminated in the stools, their presence is guaranteed only by daily replenishment.

Bacteria and yeasts are supplied in slight amounts on the skins of fruits, seeds, and vegetables. The same bacteria and yeasts have been considerably concentrated from wheat or rye, in a sourdough, and some of them do survive and thrive in the bread after baking. Naturally fermented milks, such as those made in Sweden, Finland, and the Middle East, are rich sources of these favorable lactic bacteria. Commercial yogurts frequently contain a man-made selection of bacteria similar to that found in the natural ferments for milk. Pasteurized versions of any of these will have greatly reduced quantities of favorable bacteria. All the various ethnic fermented foods, including tempeh, natto from soybeans, and fermented vegetables, such as sauerkraut cabbage, generously supply beneficial bacteria. The realization of how important the healthy growth of bacteria in the colon is has led to new commercialized preparations of bacteria, known as probiotics. Probiotics populate the colon with good bacteria, and are the opposite of antibiotics, which tend to destroy large numbers of colonic bacteria. (Prebiotics are the soluble fibers required for this favorable bacterial growth.) An absence of beneficial bacteria in the colon can lead to diarrhea just as surely as an overgrowth of unfavorable bacteria can. In either case, a good way to keep the colon healthy is to consume a natural probiotic, such as yogurt, or a commercial probiotic preparation, along with a diet that includes a plentiful supply of soluble fiber.

Feeding the Bacteria for a Healthy Colon

Lactic bacteria thrive in milk because they use the milk sugar, lactose, built from two sugar molecules—glucose and galactose. Plant fibers are polymers made up from numerous kinds of simple sugars, including glucose and galactose, so lactic bacteria from fermented milks can often make good use of plant fiber for food. Each type of bacteria tends to favor the use of a particular group of sugars, with the result that the many kinds of bacteria in the colon can thrive together. In order to survive, the bacteria must be fed, and the various types of dietary fiber favor different groups of bacteria. For the predominating bifidobacteria, the food source of choice seems to be the oligosaccharides, with short chains of sugar molecules.

The oligosaccharides, with fructose predominating (oligofructose), appear to be important. In a study, a group of volunteers eating a strictly controlled diet was first fed a dose of white sugar daily for two weeks, and were then fed the same amount of oligofructose daily for the next two weeks. During the sucrose feeding, their bifidobacteria count dropped dramatically to 17 percent of the total, and was replaced by unfavorable bacteria. Then, after taking the oligofructose, the bifidobacterial count rose to a very healthy 82 percent of the total. This new discovery has been commercialized, and oligosaccharides have been named prebiotics, and are the food for the probiotic bifidobacteria.

Oligosaccharides, naturally present in whole-plant foods, such as the oligofructose from artichoke, asparagus, banana, garlic, leek, onion, and wheat, have been studied, but oligosaccharides seem to be well distributed in many other whole-plant foods that have yet to be studied. The varied fibers from natural whole-plant foods, including oligosaccharides, are better for promoting the growth of favorable bacteria than the resistant-starch fiber produced in refined white-flour pasta or baked goods. Refined-flour baked goods do little to promote the growth of healthy bifidobacteria and lactobacillus in the colon because they provide such a small amount of fiber, even when the resistant starch is included.

The extent of the bacterial attack on fiber from whole plants will be partly governed by whether it has been eaten raw or cooked, and whether it has been finely or coarsely processed. Lignin is almost unaffected by the colonic bacteria, and since it is naturally bound to other kinds of fiber, its physical form can affect the process. Finely ground dietary fiber in the coats of seeds that contain lignin will be more readily attacked by the colonic bacteria than the coarsely ground grains and seeds, such as wheat or flaxseed.

Some of the bulk in stools is due to the presence of a plentiful amount of favorable bacteria. Excess fiber, as found in coarsely ground whole grains and seeds that have resisted bacterial attack and have good water-holding capacity, also contributes bulk, as do the fiber gums produced by the bacteria themselves. When there is an appropriate excess of fiber in the stools, bile acids are eliminated in greater quantity, which further adds to the bulk of the stools. In the presence of favorable bacteria, these excreted bile acids are harmless, but if they are degraded by the enzymes of unfavorable bacteria they can become carcinogens. The presence of a high percentage of beneficial bacteria in the colon is manifested by the following: daily, easy elimination after the food has transited the system for only one or two days; high acidity of the stools; a favorable cholesterol profile as a result of absorption of the short-chain fatty acids; and generally good health and immunity.

PART TWO

Fiber in History and Disease Prevention

4

Plant Foods through the Ages

Many books have been written on the history of foods. A few highlights of this history show how high-fiber foods have been used, and how the consumption of fiber has declined dramatically over the centuries, and at a speeded-up rate in the past two hundred years. Some concepts in this chapter are so crucial to understanding the value of fiber in health that we will look at them again from different points of view in other chapters.

Before Agriculture Began

There are ancient petroglyphs (line carvings on rocks) in the desert canyons of northern Nevada and other parts of the West that depict how Native Americans went into forests in the canyons near Reno to pick berries, leaves, and nuts. In the Southwest, Native Americans ate grains and beans and the nutritious stems of bulrushes.

Before the era of agriculture, people in the temperate regions gathered leaves, nuts and other seeds, roots, and stems, and made these a major part of their diet. Today these foods are called unrefined whole foods.

In these temperate climates, the animals that early people killed for food were eaten together with the unrefined whole-plant foods. The digestive systems of humans and other closely related primates (the ape families) required sufficient plant fibers to function properly. The human digestive system is different from that of meat-eating animals. Those animals, humans included, who eat a more plant-based diet (with meat forming only a part of it) have a long digestive tract. The small intestine is twenty feet long and one inch in diameter. The large intestine (colon) is another five or six feet in length, and about two inches in diameter. The plant food stays in the system long enough to be fermented by bacteria and yeasts, an essential part of the digestion process. Animals that eat meat only have a short digestive tract and most of the meat is completely digested, leaving very little residue to be fermented, and therefore only small firm stools to be eliminated. Although dogs and their wolf relatives are meat eaters in the wild, they are known to relish the stomach of their prey (usually a grass-eating animal) because they know instinctively that it is full of grasses and other fibrous foods needed to help keep their own digestive systems clean.

Coprolites Reveal Fiber Consumption over Millennia

The consumption of fiber over millennia has been studied using coprolites, which are ancient dried stools, some dating back 10,000 years. In the 1970s, these markers were found in Western deserts by Dr. M. Klicks and other researchers, and when analyzed, they revealed the high-fiber intake of ancient people, and the tremendous decline in fiber intake over the centuries.

Figure 4.1, derived from Klicks' data, illustrates this dramatic decline in fiber intake. It confirms that, for 99 percent of the span of human existence,

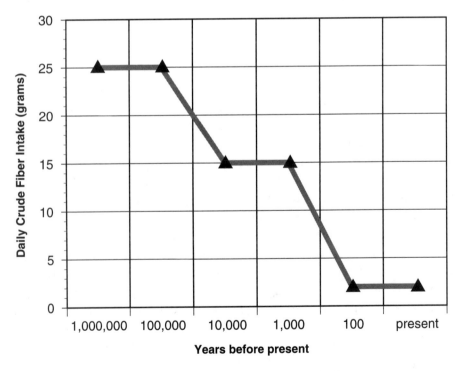

Figure 4.1. Decline in Fiber Intake through the Ages

the human digestive system was exposed to a diet that supplied high levels of the plant foods that make the digestive system work efficiently to eliminate residues from the body and prevent constipation and its consequences. Since this graph is from data gathered before current methods of analysis were developed, it uses crude fiber values, but that is not as important as its graphic depiction of the change over the years.

The Agricultural Era

As the era of agriculture began, grains and other small seeds became more and more the foundation of the human diet in many climates. Native grains were consumed as whole grains. Small grains, such as the quinoa of the Incas in Peru, the amaranth of the Aztecs and the Mayas, the teff of the Ethiopians, the blue corn of the Anasazi in the southwestern United States, the barley, rye, and wheat of Europe, and the rice of Asia, were never refined in the early days of agriculture.

Stone mills later used to grind barley and wheat were found in twentieth-century excavations among the ruins of major cities in the Roman Empire—Pompeii, Herculaneum, and other cities in southern Italy that had been preserved for centuries under the volcanic lava that had covered them during the eruption of Mount Vesuvius near Naples in 79 A.D. These excavated mills ground very coarse flour to make bread. The peasants ate the wholegrain bread, while the aristocracy sifted the flour, because white was considered the pure color. Naturally, the peasants were envious of the rich people who were eating the *pure* white flour, a concept that has survived the centuries. But the flour in Roman times, made by sifting the ground wheat through coarse sieves (made from stems of various marsh plants or papyrus), produced a very different, much less refined, flour than the highly refined white flours of today. Even as sieves become more sophisticated over the centuries, the stone mill produced flour that, even after sifting, still contained a small quantity of germ and bran.

Some stone mills have survived the introduction of roller milling, the current refining method. During a visit to a commercial mill in a small village in central Italy several years ago, the owner mentioned that, although he has both stone mills and roller mills, he was eating only the flour from his stone mill because every day he noticed how much was removed from the white flour produced by his roller mills. In America, although increasing numbers of companies are preparing stone-ground, wholegrain flours for specialty markets, these flours have not yet reached the majority of the population.

5

Fiber and Health through the Ages

The Chronology of Fiber

In the fourth century B.C., Hippocrates, considered by many to be the father of medicine, stressed the value of wholegrain flour to help keep the bowel (large intestine, or colon) healthy.

The idea that sifted, purified, or refined foods are desirable goes back millennia. The Roman aristocracy preferred sifted white flour and left the dark flour for the peasants. This thinking carried over to making animal products, such as meats—usually very concentrated sources of protein and fat—the *foundation* of the diet. Some nutritionists define this as making meat the *center* of the plate. Most restaurants serve a large piece of meat or fish, with a few vegetables beside it, and white bread; white pasta, even if made from hard, high-protein wheat, is the only pasta choice—wholegrain pastas and breads, which are loaded with flavor and nutritional value, are almost never on the menu. This is a carryover from the low-fiber, high-meat diet of the aristocracy of antiquity, which was viewed with great envy by the poor bean eater, who was, ironically, lean compared to the overweight aristocracy.

In the ninth century A.D., a Persian physician named Hakim taught the value of fiber-rich foods for healthy bowel function. In the latter part of the fifteenth century, Thomas Tryon, a student of physics, said in his *Way to Health, Long Life and Happiness,* published in London:

"If you set any value on health, and have a mind to preserve nature, you must not separate the finest from the coarsest flour; because that which is fine is naturally of an obstructive and stopping quality; but on the contrary, the other, which is coarse, is of a cleansing and opening nature, therefore the bread is best which is made of both together. It is more wholesome, easier of digestion, and more strengthening than bread made of the finest flour . . . for when the finest flour is separated from the coarsest and branny parts, neither the one nor the other has the true operations of the wheat meal. The eating of fine breads, therefore, is inimical to health, and contrary both to nature and reason; and was at first invented to gratify wanton and luxurious persons, who are ignorant both of themselves, and the true virtue and efficacy of natural things."

The above quote was reprinted from Sylvester Graham's nineteenth-century book, *Treatise on Bread and Bread Making*. Graham went on to support the wholegrain idea, saying, ". . . the bread of a large portion of the laboring class, or peasantry, throughout Europe, Asia, and Africa, and the islands of the ocean . . . is made of the whole substance of the grain from which it is manufactured. No one who is sufficiently enlightened in physiological science to qualify him to judge correctly in this matter can doubt that bread made in the best manner from [*unsifted*] wheat meal, is far better adapted to the anatomical structure and physiological powers of the alimentary organs of man, than bread made of superfine wheat flour and consequently, the former is far more conducive to the health and vigor and general well-being of man than the latter."

In 1847, another London author, Dr. D. Carr, published his treatise, *The Necessity of Brown Bread for Digestion, Nourishment and Sound Health and the Injurious Effects of White Bread.*

In 1840, an American physician, J. Burne, wrote *A Treatise on the Causes and Consequences of Habitual Constipation,* which tells how he recommended "coarse brown bread" for the relief of constipation to a wealthy woman, and how she found immediate relief. The title of his book demonstrates how, even in those days, low-fiber diets were common for his patients, the wealthier members of society who could afford a physician.

In 1888, Dr. Thomas Allinson in London wrote *Advantages of Wholemeal Bread,* by which time, the roller-milling era had begun, making super-refined flour readily available to everyone. The flour was not only easy to make but was far more refined than the sifted flours made from the stone mills. To counter this, Dr. Allinson bought an old stone grinding mill to supply truly wholegrain flour in Britain.

In the late 1800s and early 1900s, nutritionists began to understand proteins, fats, and carbohydrates. Starting in the early 1900s, vitamins were being discovered, as were minerals. The major minerals, such as calcium, came first;

later, as more sophisticated analytical techniques were developed, came the trace minerals. This research is ongoing today, and better and better understanding of these nutrients is developing. Fiber, on the other hand, was not getting much attention paid to it by most researchers, but it is catching up now.

In the early 1900s, Arbuthnot Lane, a British surgeon, recognized the dangers of stagnant stools in the colon and recommended the *removal* of the colon, even if healthy, as a preventive measure because he had diagnosed so many diseases in the large bowels of his patients. Fortunately, he later realized that this drastic step was not necessary because bran and other vegetable fibers would keep the colon healthy.

In the 1920s, Robert McCarrison, another British physician, published his classic book, *Studies in Deficiency Diseases,* and praised the strong physique of the people of northern India, who ate a diet based on whole cereals, fruits, and vegetables. In the 1920s and '30s, the researchers G. R. Cowgill and W. E. Anderson studied wheat bran in controlled clinical studies and found it was very effective in preventing constipation and promoting proper bowel function.

In 1939, Dr. Weston A. Price published *Nutrition and Physical Degeneration,* in which he described his worldwide research on populations in many regions who ate the foods of their ancestors. Price, a dentist, photographed the teeth and jaw structure of indigenous people around the world, which graphically showed that people born of parents who ate the ancestral diet had a much better facial structure than people who ate a diet of refined grains.

Between 1939 and 1945, during World War II, when flour in England was either unrefined or less refined, there was a decline in the death rate from major diseases, such as heart disease.

In the late 1960s and early 1970s, the fiber hypothesis was born. Sir Richard Doll encouraged Drs. Burkitt and Trowell to pursue it as the cause of many diseases. At the same time, Dr. Alexander Walker's studies in South Africa suggested the value of higher fiber intake.

In 1975, a forgotten fiber pioneer, Surgeon Captain T. L. Cleave, published his ideas about refined carbohydrates and disease in his now-classic book, *The Saccharine Disease: Conditions Caused by the Taking of Refined Carbohydrates, Such as Sugar and White Flour."*

On July 14, 1976, Dalhousie University in Halifax, Nova Scotia, hosted one of the first international meetings on fiber. Key people in fiber research, including Denis Burkitt, got together for the first time, and the *Proceedings* of the meeting were published.

Between 1975 and 1980, the fiber era was born in earnest. Books were published by fiber experts Denis Burkitt, Hugh Trowell, T. L Cleave, Gene Spiller, Neil Painter, and others, that detailed the importance of fiber and unrefined plant foods in the diet. Many research papers on fiber began to appear in scientific and medical journals.

In 1977, Trowell testified on the relationship between fiber, diet, and disease at the McGovern hearings in the United States Senate. And in 1978, the first symposium on fiber in nutrition was held at the International Congress of Nutrition in Rio de Janeiro, Brazil.

In the 1980s and 1990s, the phytochemical era was born. Phytochemicals that accompany fiber—from powerful antioxidants to tartaric acid—are found to be very protective compounds and not just colors or flavors. The terms antioxidants, phytochemicals, and phytonutrients began to appear regularly and became common words. Today, there are meetings on fiber and phytochemicals in many countries, from New Zealand to England, many books on fiber are published, and hundreds of researchers and physicians now focus on fiber and phytochemicals.

In the twenty-first century, more and more antioxidants and beneficial non-antioxidant compounds, such as tartaric acid in grapes and tamarinds, and phytic acid in grains and beans, are found to be protective. (In 2003, we published a paper in the *British Journal of Nutrition* on how fiber and tartaric acid work together.)

6

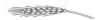

From Crude Fiber
to Dietary Fiber

The Unbelievably Long Life of the Term *Crude Fiber*

On food labels, as well as in research and analysis of fiber foods, the accepted term for fiber in food today is *dietary fiber,* but this term has only been in use since the late 1970s. Before that, the primitive term *crude fiber* was used because fiber was not considered important in health.

It is unbelievable that the term crude fiber survived from the early 1800s to the 1970s. Even in the 1900s, after scientists had discovered the value of vitamins, minerals, proteins, carbohydrates, and fats, the term crude fiber, with its negative connotation, was still being used.

Back then, the laboratory method for determining the amount of crude fiber in a food was to boil the sample in sulfuric acid, a powerful acid, and then with sodium hydroxide, a powerful alkaline substance. The substances that remained were varying percentages of what is now called dietary fiber, with some components totally lost.

Just look at a few values for some common foods and you will realize that the term crude fiber never belonged in contemporary nutrition. (*See* Figures 6.1 and 6.2.) How it survived until the late 1970s is a mystery.

Dietary Fiber, Insoluble and Soluble Fiber
Replace the Term *Crude Fiber*

In the 1970s, researchers began to realize that better methods of analysis were needed for fiber. Prior to the 1970s, food chemists and researchers David Southgate in England, Peter Van Soest and James Robertson at Cornell University, and others had used methods and terms that broke down the components of fiber and analyzed them for their components, but they were hardly ever used in nutrition studies or on food labels.

By the late 1970s and early 1980s, the term dietary fiber had entered the mainstream of nutrition and food science, due to the efforts of Hugh Trowell, David Southgate, and others in England and the United States. These scientists also made the methods of analyzing true total fiber and insoluble and soluble fiber easy enough for commercial analytical laboratories to use them routinely for thousands of foods, thereby advancing people's knowledge about fiber.

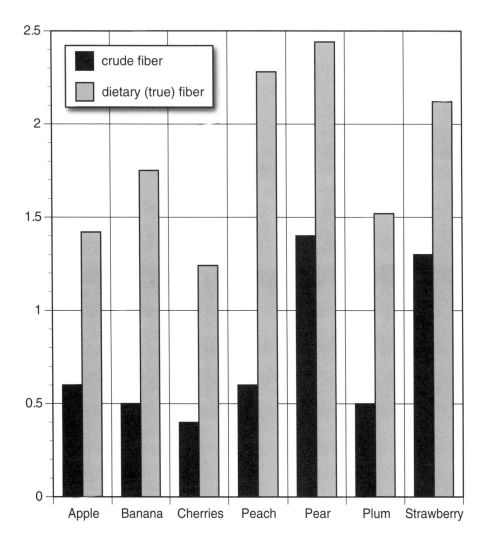

Figure 6.1. Fiber in Fruits (percent)

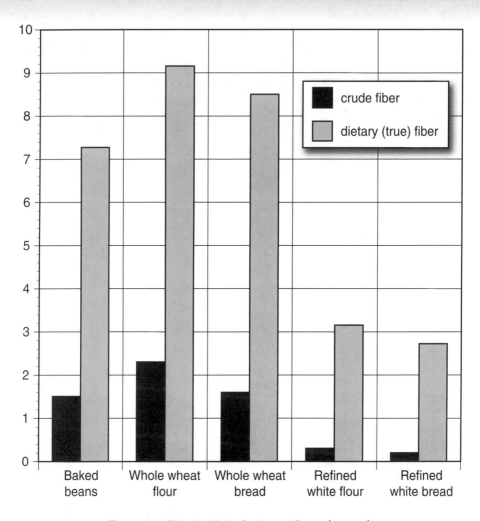

Figure 6.2. Fiber in Whole Grains and Beans (percent)

7

Health of Isolated and Non-Western Populations

The Changing Diets of China and Japan

In recent years, as a more Westernized diet, higher in meats, fats, refined grains, and sugars, and lower in vegetables, whole grains, and beans, has become popular in Japanese cities, the frequency of coronary artery disease has rapidly increased. The same is true in China, where some Western foods are replacing the simple, original Chinese dishes.

As Japanese people move from Japan to Hawaii and the continental United States and their second generation grows up on a Western diet, their rate of heart disease begins to rival that of native-born Americans.

The Republic of Seychelles—From Local to Western Diet

A good example of Westernization is found in the Republic of Seychelles, a group of islands in the Indian Ocean. After an international airport was opened there in 1971, tourism became a major industry. And with it have come Western dietary habits. As the Western diet has slowly penetrated these islands, the levels of cholesterol and heart disease in the native people have increased.

Isolated Swiss Populations

As previously mentioned, in 1939, a dentist named Weston Price published the results of his extensive worldwide travels where he studied how the health of isolated populations compared to that of the Western industrialized countries of that time. He learned that the children in the Swiss Loetschental valley, whose diet consisted mainly of whole rye bread and locally made cheeses, had very strong bodies. In a long, arduous journey to the isolated settlement of Gratchen on the Mattervisp River in the vicinity of the Matterhorn, a majestic peak on the border of Switzerland and Italy, he again found very strong, healthy people eating a diet based on whole rye bread baked in a community oven. Price recalled seeing a sixty-two-year-old woman carrying an enormous load of rye on her back at that 5,000-feet altitude. She was taking it to be ground, as it had been for centuries, in a hand mill. The people in Ayer, another village in a Swiss valley, lived on rye and local milk, often goat milk, and they too were very healthy.

Early Peruvian and Ethiopian Populations

Very small grains were the staple food in the diet for the indigenous people in both Peru and Ethiopia. These small grains—quinoa in Peru and teff in Ethiopia—were always eaten with all their fiber intact. Injera, the classic flat, pancake-like bread of Ethiopia, is now often served in American restaurants, but it is prepared with just a little teff and a lot of refined flour, as often happens when ancient grain foods move into regions where Western diets predominate.

An Endless List

The above are just a few examples of what happens when people change from a whole-plant-food diet to a refined-food diet, but the list is endless. Why should it be that a population with such technologically advanced ways of life, good education, and abundance of foods is not at the forefront of healthy eating? It is now a well-known fact that close to 80 percent of the major killer diseases, such as cancer, type-2 diabetes, and heart disease, could be prevented by diet and physical activity. Since many people have the means and the wherewithall to do so, all that is needed now is to engage their minds. It is the mind that drives all desires and choices, so a new mindset is needed before changes can take place.

Chronic Diseases Are Linked

No chronic disease lives a life of its own. Very often there are common causes that, depending on hereditary or other factors, may result in heart disease for one person, and colon cancer or diabetes for another.

8

The Reductionist's Dilemma in Food Research

What Is a Reductionist and What Is the Dilemma?

Before finding out more about how high-fiber food, or any other food component, can help to prevent disease, you need a definition to help you understand one of the great dilemmas of nutrition research, which is that nutritionists seem to contradict themselves. This is often the result of their reductionist viewpoint. Specifically, a reductionist is a scientist who searches for, and hopefully finds, one single component of food that has a definite function in the body and can prevent certain diseases or problems.

There is no doubt that reductionists are great scientists who make valuable discoveries; but when reductionism is carried to extremes, it can cause confusion in the study of nutrition and disease prevention, and lead to contradictions. This is an extremely important point and has special implications in fiber's relationship to health and disease. Taking a look at reductionism in history, will help you understand how the results of fiber research need to be interpreted.

Following the birth of chemistry as we now know it, with the discoveries of Antoine Lavoisier in the late 1700s, researchers in the 1800s and the first part of the twentieth century who were looking into the components of food and their possible relation to health and disease were able to make great discoveries. These ranged from isolating the components of proteins—the amino acids—to vitamins, minerals, and different types of fats. Isolating these factors and pinpointing their functions led to major discoveries, which helped to prevent major diseases. The discovery of niacin (vitamin B_3) and its relationship to pellagra, a digestive, skin, and nervous system disorder common in the southeastern United States and some parts of Europe, is one classic example. It was learned that refining grains, such as corn—a diet staple in those regions—removed the niacin, and this resulted in pellagra. In eastern and southern Asia, where polished rice was a staple food, it was discovered that the thiamine (vitamin B_1) lost in the polishing process that made the rice white, was causing beriberi, another serious nutritional deficiency syndrome. Finding single causes for diseases gave strength to the theory that there could be one cause for a disease, and that is how the reductionist theory got its foothold.

While it is clear that the reductionists are needed, it is also important to consider the complexity of most foods because it is generally true that benefits come mainly from the different components of food all working together to keep people healthy.

In 1922, in the early days of vitamin research, Sir Robert McCarrison wrote *Studies in Deficiency Diseases,* and concluded that, "Each vitamin is but a member of a team, and the team itself but a part of a coordinated whole." This wise statement, an important concept for the reductionist and too often forgotten by researchers now, applies equally to fiber, antioxidants, or any other nutrient.

Physical Activity and Fiber Consumption

Another type of reductionism focuses only on diet, or physical activity, or the influence of the brain. Take the case of constipation and its possible consequences on the health of the digestive system. Fiber and exercise go hand in hand here because, on a high-fiber diet, the large intestines work better if you walk, run, or do other physical activities. If the fiber is rich in antioxidants, that can help prevent damage to the cells of the large bowel, which could eventually lead to cancer of the colon, as many studies have found.

Some studies that focused only on the *amount* of fiber in foods did not show a relationship between colon cancer and fiber as did studies that looked at the overall fiber picture. Is reductionism carried to this degree good science? On the surface, it might appear so. Or is reductionism really poor science unless it is used, as it should be, as background for further studies before trying to arrive at conclusions that may influence the general public? The bottom line here is to use the reductionist techniques, but use them wisely.

9

Fiber, Colon, and Constipation

A healthy colon needs fiber and what goes with it. The colon (large intestine) begins at the end of the small intestine, where food is digested after leaving the stomach, and ends with the rectum and anus, through which stools leave the body. It is important to understand that cancer can attack the colon and rectum separately (colon cancer, rectal cancer), or together (colorectal cancer).

T. L. Cleave, a surgeon in the Royal British Navy, saw such rampant constipation in sailors during long sea voyages when there was a lack of fresh fruits and vegetables and the bread eaten was white that he fed wheat bran to those sailors, with great results. This led him to develop the hypothesis of the saccharine disease (a disease related to sugar), and to write his 1975 book of the same title.

Drs. Burkitt and Trowell, working in their hospital in Kampala, Uganda, found that the local people there had very few cases of colorectal cancer, but they did frequently find this cancer, and many other intestinal diseases, in autopsies of the British people who lived there. The same was true for diverticular disease (a condition in which pouches are formed on the wall of the intestines), and which stimulated these two physicians to develop the fiber hypothesis. Although not the first ones to praise the benefits of fiber, Burkitt and Trowell were the first ones able to attract enough attention from the medical and nutrition communities to start a new era in nutrition.

In the 1920s, John Harvey Kellogg wrote a book titled *Colon Hygiene* that praised the healthful values of wheat bran and whole grains, especially as a means of combating constipation. Soon after, in the 1930s, researchers Cowgill and Anderson published their well-controlled studies mentioned earlier showing that wheat bran was the part of the wheat that helped to insure good elimination, which helped the cereal industry to blossom.

What Is Transit Time?

Transit time refers to the time taken by food, from the time it is eaten until the undigested portion is eliminated as stools. Transit time can vary depending on the diet. In a healthy individual, it can take from one to two days. In a constipated person, transit time can be five days or more.

Various systems are used to measure transit time. In studies at our research center, we have a simple system used by many other researchers. All at one time, we have a person take forty tiny, indigestible, harmless pellets (technically known as radio-opaque pellets) that show up in an x-ray, and after every elimination we collect the stools and x-ray them, counting the number of pellets that come out each day. Transit time equals the number of days from the time the pellets are swallowed to the time they have all been expelled.

In one of our studies, an otherwise healthy young man had a transit time of over five days. He volunteered for an x-ray and all the little pellets he had swallowed were still sitting there in his colon, the ultimate sign of constipation. He got the message and quickly changed his diet after that. In the same study, just about everybody had a transit time of two days or less when the stool weight was about 200 grams (7 ounces) and below that stool weight, most transit times were longer, sometimes long enough to be reason for concern. Transit time is closely related to the weight of the stool—a bulky, softer stool moves through the colon faster and is easier to eliminate.

Transit Time, Constipation, and Diseases

Burkitt's research in the 1970s had clearly shown the relationship of transit time to stool weight in various populations and, as expected, to the kinds of diets of these populations. As he said then (and it is still true today), except for a few medical conditions, constipation can be prevented by a diet high in unrefined plant foods.

The interest in transit time and stool weight and composition grew so fast that, by the beginning of this millennium, a chapter written by professor John Cummings of the University of Dundee in Scotland for the *CRC Handbook of Dietary Fiber in Human Nutrition* contained more than forty pages of tables listing the results of studies on stool composition, transit times, stool weight, and other related data.

Disease in the Large Intestines

Today's societies have so many intestine-related conditions that books have been written about them. Some conditions and diseases related to either insufficient fiber, or insufficient accompaniments to fiber, are:

- Colon cancer;
- Constipation;
- Diverticular disease;
- Hemorrhoids;
- Rectal cancer*

Constipation Today

Things have not changed much since the late 1970s. Just walk into any drug store and look at the space taken by laxatives on the shelves of non-prescription drugs—along with painkillers, it is one of the largest. Some fiber products on that laxative shelf are safe and helpful and should not be considered laxatives, but rather fiber supplements. Still, under normal circumstances, you should try to normalize your bowel function by increasing the fiber in your diet instead of taking supplements. These may be a good alternative if you are traveling and are unable to find unrefined, whole-plant foods. Psyllium seed husk is a beneficial alternative normalizer of intestinal function, but never make a fiber supplement an excuse for not eating the right high-fiber foods.

Fiber, Exercise, and Constipation

The necessity of sufficient exercise is too often overlooked. The movement of various muscles for walking or running or almost any physical activity is crucial for proper elimination, assuming you eat enough fiber. This fiber-exercise connection is something you can easily test yourself. Do the elimination-fiber-exercise test: Eat a high-fiber diet regularly and bicycle, jog, walk, or do exercises, and soon you will feel a regular urge for proper elimination.

A division of the National Institutes of Health (NIH) that is involved with digestive diseases stressed the following important points to keep the digestive system working properly. Their key suggestions about preventing constipation confirm ours, and add other, important ones.

- Drink plenty of liquids.
- Eat a well-balanced, high-fiber diet that includes beans, bran, whole grains, fresh fruits, and vegetables.
- Exercise regularly.
- Set time aside after breakfast or dinner for undisturbed visits to the toilet. Do not ever ignore the urge to have a bowel movement.

*The most tragic of all in this part of the body.

Some situations are not related to these points, as for example some specific, serious diseases, such as a stroke (by far the most common), that may be the cause of constipation. If your constipation persists for more than a short time after you have practiced these four points, you should discuss it with a health professional.

Irritable Bowel Syndrome

This is a very common problem that is, many times, caused by a fiber deficiency. Its symptoms range from diarrhea to constipation and an unpleasant feeling in the abdomen as the colon desperately tries to do its job of eliminating waste and residues while keeping itself healthy. Dietary fiber and what goes with it can, in many cases, prevent this disease.

Many Factors Contribute to Maintaining Your Health

As you read about the interaction of fiber, physical activity, drinking enough fluids, and listening to your urge to have a bowel movement, you see how important it is to always keep in mind that the maintenance of health is the result of many interrelated factors. You also see how difficult studying the causes of diseases can be, and how important it is to use reductionism wisely in research.

10

Fiber and Cancer of the Colon and Rectum

Studies on Fiber's Role in Cancers of the Colon and Rectum

A major study on plant foods, fiber, and rectal cancer was recently published in the *American Journal of Clinical Nutrition* by Martha Slattery and other researchers from the University of Utah, together with Kaiser Permanente of Oakland, California. In analyzing possible associations between vegetables and other plant foods and cancer of the rectum in two groups, one living in Utah, the other in northern California, they found that the consumption of fruits, vegetables, and whole grains was associated with lower risk of this cancer, while a high intake of refined grains resulted in an increased risk. When the results were further analyzed for the intake of dietary fiber, the higher intakes reduced the risks more, and this was true for both men and women.

The British journal, *The Lancet,* recently published results from a major European study conducted by Sheila Bingham of the United Kingdom and a group of twenty researchers from other European countries, including Greece and Italy, on dietary fiber and its role in protection against colon cancer. This multinational study found that dietary fiber has a major protective effect against colorectal cancer when individuals who have a low-fiber intake double their fiber consumption. This protection was effective in up to 40 percent of those who previously had a low-fiber consumption, with the greatest reduction in risk seen towards the end of the colon, which is on the left side of the body.

Recent studies in the Swiss canton of Vaud and in Italy by Dr. C. LaVecchia and his colleagues, to determine the relationship between various types of fiber and the risk for colorectal cancer, were performed on people with colorectal cancer who had been admitted to the University Hospital of Lausanne. The findings were compared with people admitted for other diseases, and questionnaires about food frequency and dietary habits were used. The researchers took into account the sex, education, physical activity, and caloric intake of all those in the study, and found that the higher the total fiber intake, whether from fruits, grains, or vegetables, the lower the risk of colorectal cancer.

In an earlier Italian trial, Dr. LaVecchia studied both colon and rectal cancer in 1,953 cases admitted to Italian hospitals and, comparing them to 4,154 non-cancer controls, concluded that fiber of either fruit or vegetable origin provides additional support for the protective effect of fiber on colorectal cancer.

Dr. L. LeMarchand conducted a study among different ethnic groups in Hawaii to evaluate the role of various fibers, as well as nutrients and foods of plant origin, in the risk of colorectal cancer. The data showed that fiber from vegetables was protective.

Studies by Dr. L. McMillan and coworkers at Birmingham University in the United Kingdom showed that butyric acid—also called butyrate and produced in the colon by the fermentation of dietary fiber, along with acetic acid, also found in vinegar—may contribute to the protective effect of a high-fiber diet against colorectal cancer. These and similar acids are called short-chain fatty acids because the length of their molecule is fairly short. A common supplement, such as psyllium seed used as a bulking agent, was also found to produce butyric acid.

The complexity of colon cancer is such that not everybody agrees on which fiber or fiber food is more protective. Researcher Michael J. Hill, reviewed the scientific publications on fiber and concluded that, of all the fibers, the protective effect of cereal fiber for colorectal cancer cannot be disputed.

In Germany, Dr. W. Scheppach and associates reviewed a number of studies and concluded that excessive consumption of red meat is associated with an increased risk of colorectal cancer. In experimental cancer studies done at the same time, it was learned that protective effects resulted from consuming high-fiber carbohydrates degraded by bacteria in the colon to short-chain fatty acids.

Phytates, found in reasonable amounts in almonds and other nuts, beans, seeds, and whole grains, may have some protective properties too, according to University of Toronto Doctors M. Jenab and L. U. Thompson. Phytates are also present in smaller amounts in many other unrefined plant foods, adding to the value of their fiber content.

Many other studies support the protective effect of various fibers or high-fiber foods, either in humans or in animal tests—so many that this book could be filled just with the stories of their results. One researcher even found coffee fiber to be protective, but coffee fiber is not normally consumed.

Not All Studies Agree

The variety of fiber, fiber foods, the methods of preparation, and the difficulty in interpreting the labels of thousands of prepared foods now available in supermarkets makes fiber research very difficult, which may be the reason that a few studies did not seem to find that cereal fiber was protective. A Harvard study on nurses by Dr. Charles Fuchs and a very sophisticated research group is one example. A key observation was that the highest intake of fiber was only about 25 grams, less than an ounce a day. In our own studies, we have observed that constipation is fully relieved only when the dietary fiber intake is greater than 35 grams a day for an average-height adult. Below this level there is not enough fiber for the colon to give predictable transit times. And the same holds true for fiber's effect on disease prevention unless more than 35 grams of mixed fiber per day is consumed. The details of Dr. Fuchs' study showed that almost all the cereal fiber consumed was from refined wheat foods, containing mostly endosperm. The small proportion of fiber found in these refined wheat products is mostly resistant starch, which acts as soluble fiber and is not associated with any protective substances.

The authors evidently missed two key points. First, there was too little fiber in the diet to bring about any measurable benefit. Second, refined wheat products (white bread, white pasta, and refined cereals) containing only the endosperm of the grain lack the protective fiber from the bran and the germ.

Beyond Wheat Bran Fiber

Some studies of wheat bran, the most fibrous part of the wheat, have tried to identify specific components that may work together with all the wheat fiber. Wheat bran separated out from the whole grain was the first concentrated fiber food accepted as beneficial for preventing constipation and relieving diverticular disease.

In the late 1970s, Dr. Burkitt recommended wheat bran as a supplement because whole-wheat cereals and true whole-wheat breads are very effective for normal elimination and keeping the colon healthy. Here again, it is best not to be a reductionist and talk only about fiber, which is, after all, just one component of a food, because it has been found that two other compounds work with the fiber of wheat to make it more effective in its protective role— the oil in wheat bran and phytates.

As reported in *Cancer Research,* Bandaru S. Reddy and his associates from the American Health Foundation in Valhalla, New York, found that epidemiological (population) studies of people suggest that the higher the intake of dietary fiber, particularly fiber from cereal grains, the lower the risk for colon cancer. Reddy noted that wheat bran appears to inhibit the development of colon tumors more consistently than either oat bran or corn bran, and he attributed this to an oil in the wheat bran, which helped to lower the risk of colon cancer in the animal models he used.

The phytates present in wheat bran may also work as protectors. This collective effect shows how various foods complement each other and how a whole, natural food, such as a whole grain, should be looked at as a storehouse of many protective factors.

Why High-Fiber Foods Are Protective in Colorectal Cancer

With high-fiber foods, there is:

- A binding of cancer-producing compounds;

- A change in the concentration of different bile acids;

- Faster transit time, with faster elimination of possible cancer-producing by-products of digestive and other body functions;

- Fermentation, with production of protective compounds (butyric acid and others) that also maintain an acidic colon, which is considered a healthier colon;

- A selection of phytochemicals, such as antioxidants, oils, phytic and tartaric acids, that go with fiber;

- And probably many other phytonutrients yet to be discovered.

Fiber Increase Is a Sound Choice

Even with a few of the studies showing no protective effect by fiber, a careful overview of the research leads to the conclusion that many high-fiber foods, such as fruits, vegetables, whole wheat and other grains, and all the phytochemicals that go with them, are a good step in the prevention of colon and rectal cancer. As of now, there is not enough research on beans, but they are an intrinsic part of any plant-based, high-fiber, high-phytochemical diet. And other foods—almonds, hazelnuts, walnuts, and other nuts—add fiber to the diet as well. Because of their good protein content, they can replace some or all of the fiber-free meat proteins.

In the *European Journal of Cancer Prevention,* British researcher D. F. Evans concluded his study by saying, ". . . evidence suggests that 80–90 percent of colorectal cancers are caused by dietary and environmental factors and that the prevalence of cancer can be altered in low-risk patients by long-term alterations in dietary fiber ingestion. . . ." Sounds like a good reason to change your diet to a high-fiber, plant-based one, doesn't it?

Protect and Prevent with High Fiber

For colorectal-cancer protection and prevention, it is sound to increase high-fiber plant foods and to consider whole wheat and whole grains combined with vegetables, fruits, and beans as key parts of the diet. And it is best to vary the diet so you do not get all your fiber from just one kind of food.

11

Fiber and Diverticular Disease

The diverticula are pouches (small sacs) in the wall of the large intestine (colon) that can degenerate and become filled with contents of the colon that are supposed to be excreted. This condition can cause pain and the diverticula can rupture, resulting in a major infection if the bacteria-rich content of the colon escapes. At its worst, this disease can lead to surgery.

Diverticular disease is also called diverticulosis, and when inflammation is present, it is called diverticulitis. (The suffix *itis* is used in medicine to indicate inflammation or inflammatory disease, as in bronch*itis,* appendic*itis,* diverticul*itis.*) In diverticulitis, the sacs or pouches become filled with stool material and may become inflamed; in extreme cases, perforation of the intestinal wall or bleeding may occur.

Back in 1869, Dr. E. Klebs introduced the idea that diverticula were caused by constipation and were not something people were born with. Physicians of that era found diverticula to be a curiosity, but did not think they were a real problem until later, when it was found that if they were infected or perforated they could cause major problems, such as an infection of the region around the intestines.

This degeneration of the large intestine wall is more common in Western countries than in regions with less refined, more primitive diets high in fiber. Drs. Burkitt and Trowell discovered this in Uganda, where, as with colorectal cancer, they found a tremendous difference between their British and their Ugandan patients. There were only occasional cases in the Ugandan population, and they seldom showed up in an autopsy, but there was a much higher frequency of diverticular disease in the British residents.

It is tremendously valuable to look back to regions of Africa in the 1960s and 1970s when there was a greater chance of finding more people on unrefined, ancient diets. In 1974, after using carefully prepared questionnaires to survey over one hundred missions and rural hospitals in Africa, Dr. Trowell reported that diverticular disease was barely known in these missions and hospitals.

Researchers Neil Painter and Denis Burkitt published data in 1971 confirming that diverticular disease was rare in many countries where mostly non-refined diets were the norm. Their data included Dr. A. C. Jain's report from Zaire that he saw only one patient with the disease in nine years, and that, in 1960, Dr. J. N. Davies in Uganda reported only two cases in the 4,000 patients he had seen over fifteen years. Similar reports in the 1970s confirmed the rarity of this problem in India, Iran, Iraq, and South Africa—in 1958, Dr. K. J. Keely, reported that he had found no diverticula in 2,367 autopsies at Baragwanah Hospital. Similar rarity was found in Kenya and other African countries.

In England in the 1970s, Dr. Painter linked constipation to diverticular disease in older people who had eaten a diet low in fiber for many years, the diet referred to as a Western diet.

When the large intestines have to make a great effort to push their contents forward to be eventually expelled, the pressure inside the colon is much higher than for soft bulky stools that move along easily in the colon and are easy to eliminate. This pressure causes unnecessary and tiring straining during elimination, and can lead to secondary problems, such as hemorrhoids.

Recent Studies Supporting the Protective Effect of Fiber

Current methods, such as barium enemas, that allow x-rays of the large intestines with possible pouches, have helped the health profession study this disease in living people.

In 1980, Drs. Hyland and Taylor showed that 100 patients with diverticular disease remained free of symptoms when placed on a high-fiber diet. In 1994, W. H. Aldoori and his colleagues at the Harvard School of Public Health in Boston examined the association between dietary fiber, sources of fiber, other nutrients, and the diagnosis of diverticular disease. Analyzing data from 47,888 men in the United States, they looked into the effects of total dietary fiber and found it was protective, but found that a diet low in total dietary fiber increased the risk for the disease.

In 1998, after additional study of a large number of health professionals in the United States, and after analyzing the differences between the protective effects of different types of fiber in foods, these same researchers found that insoluble fiber, mainly cellulose, was the most effective fiber for preventing symptoms in 43,881 male health professionals from forty to seventy-five years of age. This led Dr. Aldoori's group to conclude that their findings supported the hypothesis that a diet high in dietary fiber helps prevent diverticular disease.

Monkeys are good models for fiber studies, as their digestive system is closer to humans than that of rats and other experimental animals. In one study with monkeys, the pressure inside the colon was measured after various diets. Dr. A. J. Brodribb found that the pressure was getting higher and higher as the daily fiber intake was decreased gradually from 20 to 15, 10, 5, and, finally, 0 grams. In other studies using monkeys, it was shown that diverticular disease is more frequent when a Western-type, low-fiber diet is fed than when a high-fiber diet is fed.

In 2002, Dr. Aldoori reviewed the research published between 1966 and 2002 on the prevention of diverticular disease with high-fiber diets. He concluded it is the insoluble portion of dietary fiber in high-fiber, low-fat diets that prevents this disease.

A Healthy Colon with High Fiber

High-fiber intake lowers pressure inside the colon and this helps to prevent diverticular disease. All in all, fiber helps maintain a healthy colon and rectum, and may help prevent related problems, such as hemorrhoids.

12

Fiber and Weight Control

Weight Control Beyond Looks

Excessive body weight has become an international problem. Magazine and newspaper articles talk about the overweight epidemic, and right at the root of this tragic problem is the availability of refined foods and the insufficient consumption of fiber. In the United States, the number of overweight people has grown steadily in recent years, and in Italy, the newspaper *Il Corriere della Sera* recently reported that obesity, previously unknown in Italian children, had now become a problem.

Today about 129 million American adults, age twenty and older, have excessive body weight, and of these, about 61 million are considered outright obese. A 1999–2000 survey by the National Center for Health indicates that 15 percent of children and adolescents from ages six to nineteen years, are overweight. This is doubly sad because, just thirty years ago, the number of overweight children and adolescents in the same age range was only 4–5 percent. (*See* Figure 12.1.)

The situation is just as dire for adults. Overweight is defined as moderately excessive weight, while obesity is major excessive weight when weight is compared to height. Except for just a few pounds over normal weight, both are undesirable. (*See* Figure 12.2.)

Excessive body weight is related to greater risk for many major diseases, with type-2 diabetes and heart disease at the top of the list. As you may expect, the greater the excess weight, the greater the risk. Dr. James Anderson, who has researched diabetes for many years at the University of Kentucky, states that weight management may be one of the most important steps for most obese adults with diabetes. He and his associates carefully reviewed the published research on the correlation between excessive weight and dia-

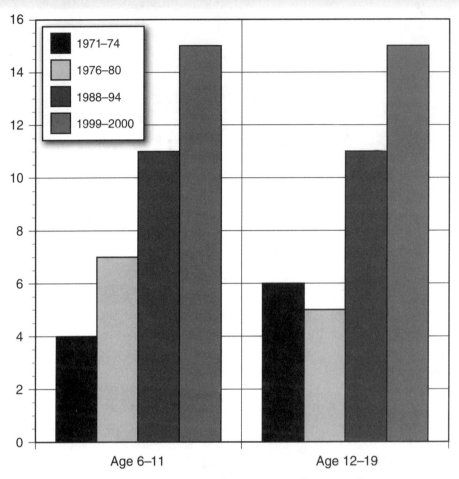

Figure 12.1. Percentage of Overweight Adolescents 1976–2000

betes, and confirmed that obesity is indeed a major contributor to the development of this disease, while weight loss by overweight people with diabetes helps to control their fasting blood sugar.

Dr. Anderson reminds us that obesity and weight gain can increase the risk for diabetes over ninety-fold, and about sixfold for diseases of the arteries that feed the heart muscle (coronary arteries from which the name coronary heart disease is derived).

And reductionism doesn't work here either because it is important to combine high-fiber, whole-plant-based diets with adequate exercise. It makes sense, and should be obvious, that eating foods with no residues reaching the colon contributes to weight gain more than high-fiber foods, and does not

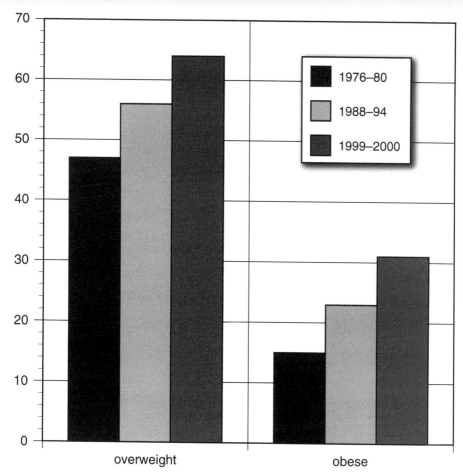

Figure 12.2. Percentage of Overweight and Obese Adults 1976–2000

give the feeling of satiety that high-fiber foods provide. That is why, although extracts and juices have a great place in a healthy diet, *they should not replace* high-fiber foods.

The Difficulties in Losing Weight

Anyone whose excess weight is more than a few pounds can tell you that losing weight is a difficult job. Just look at the large number of advertisements for weight-loss products, the enormous popularity of weight-loss books, and the growing numbers of desperate people who find drastic stomach surgery the only workable option. Extreme weight-loss diets have, it is true, found success, at least temporarily, but the real solution is to *prevent* excessive weight gain. No matter what a person's weight is, going on a high-fiber, plant-based diet and avoiding refined plant foods, makes total sense as a means of achieving a healthy, normal weight.

A Major 2003 Study Supports the Role of Whole Grains in Weight Control

A 2003 study by researchers Simin Liu, Walter C. Willett, and their associates at Brigham and Women's Hospital and Harvard Medical School, focused on whole grains as a key step in weight control. Considering that a diet high in fiber and whole grains is often recommended—even in the controversial Atkins diet, which severely restricts carbohydrates, *wholegrain* bread is allowed—these researchers felt it was important to see if an association could be found between the intake of dietary fiber and whole- or refined-grain products and long-term weight gain.

They studied 74,091 U.S. female nurses, thirty-eight to sixty-three years of age, free of major chronic diseases, and followed them from 1984 to 1996. Very careful review was made of the nurses' diets in 1984, 1986, 1990, and 1994, using special food-frequency questionnaires. Those who consumed more whole grains consistently weighed less than those who consumed fewer whole grains. The lower the intake of high-fiber foods, the greater the weight gain. Also, the greater the intake of refined grains, the greater the weight gain. This shows how completely off-base it is to talk about low-carb or high-carb breads or cereals because the only distinctions that count are whole grains or refined grains. And between these, there appears to be no doubt that the wholegrain products are an aid in weight control.

An Easy Test

If you are somewhat overweight and generally healthy, try replacing all the refined-grain products you eat with wholegrain products, eating plenty of fresh vegetables and fruit, and generally shifting to a high-fiber, low-animal-product diet. Follow your weight for about three months and see the results.

13

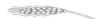

Fiber and Diabetes

What Is Diabetes?

Diabetes is basically a sugar disease. Childhood diabetes, known as type 1 or juvenile, is related more to genetics than diet. Type-2 diabetes, formerly known as adult-onset diabetes, on the other hand, is generally associated with overweight to the extent that obese people with diabetes can often manage their disease with weight loss alone.

The key hormone insulin is secreted by the pancreas as a response to sugars in the blood—sugars that may come from sugar itself or from the production of sugar after the digestion of starch. In the bodies of people with type-2 diabetes, insulin is not doing its job to help move glucose, the main sugar after digestion, into the cells, and as a result, insulin injections or other treatments may have to be employed. There are a number of causes for this, but whatever the cause, type-2 diabetes and overweight go hand in hand in most cases.

A Rare Disease in the Africa of the 1930s

It is fascinating to see how so many health problems and diseases are typical of refined-plant-food diets and urban living patterns, from colon cancer to diverticulosis, constipation, diabetes, heart disease, and obesity. When Dr. Hugh Trowell began to treat patients in Nairobi, Kenya, in the 1930s, diabetes was extremely rare in African blacks. Today, however, diabetes has penetrated East Africa, and is widespread in Westernized countries all over the world.

Diabetes for All Ages in the United States

In America, more than 18 million people, over 6 percent of the population, have diabetes of some kind. The Center for Research in Disease Prevention estimates that about 13 million cases are diagnosed, with more than 5 million undiagnosed. Many of these people have type-2 diabetes, which can be prevented with proper diet and sufficient exercise.

Flour in Europe during World War II and Diabetes

In Europe, flour, and the bread made from it during World War II and in the postwar years (1942 to 1953), had a mandatory higher fiber content. Called the "national flour," it was less refined, which resulted in a greatly increased consumption of grain fiber, up to six-fold.

In England, Dr. Trowell found that the deaths from type-2 diabetes, which had been lower during the war years and in the late 1940s, began to slowly rise from the mid-1950s onward. One of the main reasons was that, as white flour became available again, the higher fiber mandate for flour was relaxed and people quickly changed to it because wholegrain flour reminded them of the war years. This happened in Italy and other European countries where, during the war, the flour used to make bread had to be less sifted, and the rich and poor alike welcomed the return of sifted white flour as a sign of normal times.

Diabetes in the New Millennium

Based on experience with his patients and on his careful review of the literature (he cites more than 100 scientific papers published in the 1980s and '90s), Dr. James Anderson, a diabetes expert at the University of Kentucky, reached several conclusions:

1. Dietary fiber is extremely useful in the treatment of diabetes.

2. Although more work was needed to confirm the prevention of type-2 diabetes, much evidence pointed to dietary changes considered valuable in preventing diabetes.

Another major researcher in this field at the University of Toronto, Dr. David Jenkins found long-term benefits from using high-carbohydrate, high-fiber diets, in both insulin-dependent and non-insulin-dependent diabetes.

In 1999, Dr. Laura Lockwood studied Hispanic-American Seventh-Day Adventists who ate a plant-based diet high in fiber carbohydrates, and compared them to Hispanic-American Catholics, who ate a regular Western diet that was not plant-based and was low in fiber. The Seventh-Day Adventists had lower blood pressure, lower weight, lower fasting blood sugar (glucose) and insulin, lower cholesterol and blood fats (triglycerides), and a higher concentration of good HDL cholesterol when compared to the Catholics. This diet study is a reminder that a true plant-based diet is also lower in animal products so it is important to look at the entire diet.

In 2001, at the Children's Hospital Medical Center in Cincinnati, Ohio, Dr. H. J. Kalkwarf found that when their intake of fiber was higher, pregnant women with type-1 diabetes required lower amounts of the insulin that is a part of their daily life. This suggests that health professionals should encourage a higher intake of dietary fiber to control blood-sugar concentrations, including pregnant women with diabetes.

In 2002, an Italian researcher, Dr. R. Giacco, showed that dietary fiber controls blood-sugar levels and other aspects of diabetes. In people with diabetes, he found that dietary fiber decreases their blood-sugar levels, their insulin, and blood fat concentrations, and has a cholesterol-lowering effect. Equally important, his research showed that these effects continued for a long time.

A Disease That Can Be Prevented in Most Cases

For most people, type-2 diabetes can be prevented. A high-fiber, whole-plant-food diet, combined with sufficient physical activity and a moderate intake of high-fat foods, is the key to this prevention. Just as it does for constipation, fiber triumphs here too.

14

Fiber, Heart Disease, and Cholesterol

The Number-One Killer in Western Countries

Heart disease is a main cause of death in the Western world. What is intriguing is that, as far back as 1974, Dr. G. Rose showed that, in different Western countries studied, deaths from heart disease and colon cancer were related. This supports the concept that these two major deadly diseases are influenced by people's way of life, with improper diet and lack of exercise as the primary causes.

In 2001, more than 900,000 Americans died of cardiovascular disease, accounting for about 39 percent of all deaths. Remember that coronary heart disease is a disease of the arteries that feed the heart muscle. If the coronary arteries lose their flexibility (arteriosclerosis) and become clogged by deposits of plaques (atherosclerosis) and then are blocked for whatever reason—for instance, by a blood clot that gets caught in a narrowed artery—major heart problems will result, such as pain (angina), a heart attack, or possibly, even death.

Heart Disease in Africa

During their work in Africa, Drs. Burkitt and Trowell found that heart disease was rare in rural communities and cities except for the most Westernized population, the British subjects who ate a diet similar to their diet in England. And Dr. Alexander Walker reported that the Bantu people of South Africa, who consumed a diet high in grain fiber, had very few cases of coronary heart disease.

Soluble-Fiber and Highly Soluble-Fiber Products Are Protective

In people with high blood cholesterol, a large number of studies have shown that the addition to the diet of gums and other, similar soluble-fiber products lowers their blood cholesterol. This fact has been proven so many times that it leaves no doubt as to the efficacy of such fibers. Since a high cholesterol equals a greater risk of coronary heart disease, it is important for the diet to supply enough of these soluble fibers.

The Los Angeles Atherosclerosis Study

At the University of Southern California (USC), Dr. Huiyun Wu studied the effect of dietary fiber and the progression of atherosclerosis, deadly deposits in the arteries, in the Los Angeles area, and he published the results in 2003. The study followed 269 women between forty-five and sixty years old, and 304 men, between forty and sixty, who did not have a history of heart attacks or strokes. They were followed for three years, with information gathered in the beginning, halfway through, and at the end of the study.

The intake of dietary fiber, soluble fiber (including pectin), and insoluble fiber was studied in order to find out if there was a connection with the development of arterial deposits that could eventually be deadly. The study looked at all kinds of factors that could affect the development and progress of atherosclerosis, such as smoking, exercise, and caloric, fat, and cholesterol intake. Pectin is very high in many fruits and vegetables and is actually produced for commercial use from fruits, such as apples. This study unearthed a small but significant relationship between total fiber, soluble fiber (pectin), and HDL cholesterol levels: the greater the intake of fiber, soluble fiber, or pectin, the higher the good HDL level.

Jenkins' "Garden of Eden" Diet Study

In a 2003 review, Dr. David Jenkins writes about heart disease in the kind of non-reductionist approach that is so crucial in preventing chronic diseases. He defines the "Garden of Eden" diet as a plant-based diet, naturally high in fiber, plant proteins, and phytochemicals, which is key in preventing heart disease and in reducing the need for drug therapy to lower blood cholesterol. He defines this diet as "high in dietary fiber, vegetable protein, plant sterols, and associated phytochemicals, and low in saturated and trans-fatty acids." Dr. Jenkins and his associates fed a group of people a plant-food diet that was high in nuts, leafy vegetables, and fruits. The result was that the healthy people in the study had their blood cholesterol lowered as much by this diet as by medication. Again, this study is about high-fiber foods and all the other great nutrients and phytochemicals that go with them.

Soluble Fibers Lower Cholesterol

As far back as 1995, researcher Stewart Truswell, reviewing studies carried out up to that time, found that all the soluble fibers—guar gum, oat bran, pectin, and psyllium—repeatedly demonstrated a blood-cholesterol-lowering effect.

In a 1997 Stanford University study, Drs. Christopher Jensen, William Haskell, and James Whittam confirmed the blood-cholesterol-lowering effect of a mixture of guar gum, locust bean gum, pectin, and psyllium seed, when people were given 15 grams a day of this mixture.

Oat Studies

Oatmeal, whole oats, cracked oats, and oat bran lower blood cholesterol. After extensive scrutiny of the available research on the subject, the U.S. Food and Drug Administration (FDA) has allowed cereal companies to make a cholesterol claim for oat products on their labels. Whole oats contain beta-glucan, a type of soluble fiber that appears to be the blood-cholesterol-lowering component of oats. In 1990, our center conducted a study in which people with high blood cholesterol consumed oats or guar gum, and both foods lowered their cholesterol levels. Many subsequent studies confirmed that oats and oat bran do lower blood cholesterol.

Rice Bran

A 1998 study by Dr. Ann L. Gerhardt shows that some of the non-fiber components of a food are also important and that, with a high-fiber food like rice bran, there is more in that food than fiber that is active in lowering cholesterol. The study compared rice bran, which contains rice bran oil, to oat bran, which contains soluble fiber and is now accepted as a food that lowers blood cholesterol. When the rice bran was given to people with high cholesterol for six weeks, their blood cholesterol and harmful low-density lipoprotein (LDL) cholesterol went down.

Konjac Mannan

The researcher Dr. Hsaio-Ling Chen gave people with type-2 diabetes, who are at a higher risk for heart disease than people without diabetes, powdered konjac mannan. The konjac is a tuber, an underground stem similar to the potato, that usually produces buds from which a new plant will develop. It contains a high concentration of glucomannan, a type of soluble fiber, which is extracted, dried, and either used in food products or made into a powder supplement. After twenty-eight days of taking fairly low amounts of the konjac fiber, the people in the study had their total blood cholesterol lowered by 11 percent, their bad LDL cholesterol fell by 21 percent, and the bile acid in their stools, which is considered a possible mechanism for cholesterol lowering, was increased. Blood-sugar levels also fell, confirming that these good fibers help in more ways than one.

Rhubarb Fiber Also Lowers Blood Cholesterol

In 1997, Dr. V. Goel showed the cholesterol-lowering effects of a fiber prepared from rhubarb stalk in men with high blood cholesterol. The preparation he used contained about 66 percent insoluble fiber and 8 percent soluble fiber.

Bean Fiber Plus Bean Protein Is Protective

In 2001, Dr. L. A. Bazzano and her colleagues at Tulane University in New Orleans, in conjunction with researchers at the NIH, concluded that an increased intake of legumes could be an important part of a dietary approach to the prevention of heart disease in American men and women. These researchers felt that the protective effect is probably due both to the bean protein and the water-soluble fiber of beans. Their study involved 9,632 men and women in a large national nutrition and health study. When those who ate beans four or more times a week were compared to those who ate beans less than once a week, their risk for coronary artery disease was 22 percent lower than those who consumed fewer beans.

The Cocoa Bran Study

In 2000, Dr. David Jenkins at the University of Toronto published the results of a cocoa-bean bran study done with a chocolate-flavored breakfast cereal in the *Archives of Internal Medicine.* Since it is well known that beans help reduce the risk for heart disease and help keep the colon healthy, he studied the bran, the outside layer, of the cocoa bean. He found that it not only increased stool weight, as might be expected, but it also helped protect against cholesterol oxidation—oxidized cholesterol is more harmful that non-oxidized cholesterol. In addition, the cocoa bran also raised the good HDL cholesterol.

Fiber and Syndrome X

Syndrome X is a group of conditions associated with insulin resistance, which means that insulin, a key hormone in body function, cannot do its job properly. This results in an increased risk of coronary heart disease and strokes. In 2003, the researcher B. M. Davy reviewed the literature and found study results showing that fiber was protective when 25–35 grams of it were consumed daily.

The Diabetes—Heart Disease Link

Since type-2 diabetes makes people more susceptible to heart disease, some studies have looked at the effects of fiber on both diseases. At the University of North Carolina, Dr. M. McIntosh found that food rich in soluble fiber, and consumed at a fairly high level (50 grams of total fiber that was about half soluble) had improved blood sugar and blood cholesterol levels compared to people who consumed half as much fiber (25 grams of fiber with the same 50 percent of soluble fiber). This points out that 25 grams of fiber a day is not enough.

Fruits and Vegetables Are Protective

In a collaborative study by four universities—Boston University, University of Minneapolis, University of Utah, and Washington University—Dr. Luc Djoussé and other researchers found that the consumption of fruits and vegetables is related to lower levels of bad LDL cholesterol in both men and women. Whether it is the fiber, what goes with it, or most likely, both working together, is still an open question for the researcher. For everyone else, the importance of consuming more fruits and vegetables, and adding more whole grains and beans to the diet is obvious.

The Protection of High–Fiber Food Is Now Well Established

In a 2002 article in the *Journal of the American Medical Association,* researchers F. B. Hu and Walter Willett wrote about reviewing many research publications on the subject of high-fiber foods. They found overall that one recommended step should be a diet high in whole grains, fruits, and vegetables, and low in refined grains.

15

Fiber, Breast Cancer, and Other Diseases

Breast Cancer—Possible Protection by Fiber?

The connection between high-fiber foods and the protective effects of fiber needs more study. First of all, there is a need to focus on whole foods high in fiber and all the other protective phytochemicals. Since it is well known that these high-fiber foods tend to be protective, they should be part of a general cancer-protective diet. A few major studies are worth looking at.

Breast Cancer in an Italian Study

In 1997, researcher C. LaVecchia reviewed breast-cancer cases in many medical centers in Italy. He analyzed the relationship between various fibers and breast-cancer risk in 2,569 women with medically-confirmed breast cancer. Using sophisticated statistical methods, he then looked at 2,588 women admitted to the same hospitals for acute non-cancer, non-hormone-related diseases. The results of this large study suggested that fiber intake—both insoluble cellulose and soluble fibers—may give some protection against breast cancer. Again, in 1998, LaVecchia reviewed the published research on breast cancer and fiber and concluded that some studies show protection by a high intake of high-fiber foods, while others do not. He feels this is most likely due to the many different types of fiber in the different populations.

These conflicting results found by LaVecchia and others show that fiber foods contain many different types of fiber and many phytochemicals, and that they may be prepared in many different ways, from raw to cooked, or as part of recipes that may also include either animal or vegetable fat, which would diminish their effectiveness. These breast cancer results confirm the need to eat a variety of foods high in fiber from vegetables, fruits with their soluble fiber, and whole grains with cellulose in their bran.

Other Diseases

The major diseases and the possible protection against them provided by fiber and a high-fiber diet has now been covered. It is resoundingly clear that high-fiber foods may help prevent many of them, and it is possible to conclude that dietary fiber and what goes with it can also be protective for other diseases and health problems, such as prostate cancer, and reduced immunity.

The Plus-and-Minus Principle

The plus-and-minus principle is a key to any changes in your eating program and applies to most of the diseases discussed.

When researchers study how diet relates to health and illness in various populations and regions of the world, they find it is generally true that a diet high in beans, fruits, whole grains, and vegetables is also low in animal products. A diet in which olive oil is the main oil, for example, is often a diet in which this oil has replaced a saturated animal fat in food preparation or on your bread. This means that an addition equals a subtraction or, you could say, a plus for one food equals a minus for another.

For ideal results, when changing eating patterns it is important to create a new balance of foods by decreasing the use of animal products and adding more unrefined, whole-plant foods supplemented by juices and teas.

16

What the Medical and Nutrition Experts Currently Think about Fiber

In this chapter, well-known experts in medicine and nutrition share their thinking on fiber and high-fiber diets. These excerpts from interviews with them give a better understanding of the value of fiber and phytochemicals.

James W. Anderson, M.D.
Professor of Medicine and Clinical Nutrition, University of Kentucky
Director, HMR Weight Management Program, University of Kentucky
President, Obesity Research Network

When Denis Burkitt started talking about fiber, he talked about colon cancer. And colon cancer was at the top of the list for a long time. There were three studies that raised questions about that. But I think that fiber still has protective effects against colon cancer and that we are talking about foods rich in fiber with what I call the *fellow travelers,* the phytonutrients that you have discussed in this book and that have major protective effects. I think with colon cancer there is still good evidence that fiber intake is protective from colon cancer.

Hugh Trowell got into the metabolic diseases and he talked about diabetes and coronary heart disease. I think there is good evidence that fiber fights five major conditions:

- Diabetes
- Gastrointestinal (digestive) disorders
- Heart disease
- Hypertension
- Obesity

There is good evidence that fiber is protective from coronary heart disease. We have done statistical reviews, what statisticians call *meta-analyses* in this area, and nutrition-wise fiber is the strongest protector from coronary heart disease that we know of. High-fiber intake reduces risk of coronary heart disease by about 30 percent.

Fruits and vegetables are the good protectors. Fruit consumption results in about a 10-percent reduction and vegetables in about a 15-percent reduction. Whole grains reduce the risk for coronary heart disease about 30 percent, almost as much as dietary fiber.

These are population studies, what we call epidemiological or observational studies, but there have been about three studies documenting that high-fiber diets are protective.

If we move to diabetes, there are limited observational studies that fiber protects from diabetes. There are several clinical studies showing that high-fiber intake is associated with lower risk for diabetes. There is evidence that low-fat diets protect from diabetes and also evidence that low-glycemic-index foods, foods that do not cause a major rise in blood sugar after consuming them, protect from diabetes, as well as some evidence that high-fiber diets protect from diabetes.

Hypertension is interesting. Most of what we have with hypertension are observational or clinical trials. And you know we have the DASH (dietary approaches to stop hypertension) diet that lowers blood pressure, but also there are a large number of studies showing that increased fiber intake decreases blood pressure. Again, this may be related to the phytonutrients that go along with fiber—potassium and magnesium would be the major ones, but phospholipids may also contribute to improvement in blood pressure. So I think there is pretty good evidence that fiber is protective from high blood pressure.

There is a fair amount of epidemiology that fiber protects from obesity, and no evidence that contravenes this. Again, though, epidemiology leads to clues, but is not definitive. A number of clinical trials show that increasing fiber intake, even increasing fiber supplements, aids in weight loss, so there is a fair amount of data here. In addition, fiber increases the feeling of fullness. We are now learning there is a whole array of digestive hormones with names most people have never heard before, such as CCK, GIV, GLP1, glucagon, PYY, and others that are beneficially affected by dietary fiber.

I have talked about prevention of disease, but the role of fiber in the treatment of disease would start with blood cholesterol and triglycerides, the basic fats in the blood. Soluble fiber specifically helps to decrease cholesterol and triglycerides. The most potent soluble fiber for this is psyllium, followed by oat bran or oat gum, then other water-soluble fibers, such as guar gum. These soluble fibers lower the LDL cholesterol, the bad cholesterol, specifically, which is probably how they contribute to reducing the risk for coronary heart disease.

High-fiber intakes lower triglycerides. One of the enigmas of increased carbohydrate intake is that an increased amount of carbohydrate *without* fiber can *raise* the triglycerides. Not long ago, we had a major statistical review—a meta-analysis as discussed above—that shows how effective high-fiber diets are. In our research here, we did one study in people with diabetes and another in people without diabetes, and in both studies, a high-carbohydrate, high-fiber diet lowered triglycerides. (The best way to reduce blood triglycerides is with a low-fat, high-fiber diet.)

Fiber slows stomach emptying and evens out the rise in blood sugar after a meal. In diabetes, fibers act to increase insulin-sensitivity (insulin is a key hormone in sugar utilization). Making the body more sensitive to insulin reduces the need for insulin and helps people stay off the medicine intended to reduce their dosage of insulin or diabetes medication. So fibers provide a lot of health benefits for people with diabetes.

Increasing fiber intake will lower blood pressure, and I think high-fiber intakes are part of our treatment for obesity. High-fiber diets are more filling, they increase the feeling of satiation, which means they decrease hunger between meals. High-fiber foods have fewer calories per ounce of food and they also have favorable effects on hormones in the digestive system, so fibers have many ways of acting therapeutically in obesity.

Here we use fiber therapy for digestive diseases. Fiber promotes regularity and it has a role in irritable bowel syndrome—maybe 20 to 25 percent of the population has irritable bowel syndrome with abdominal pain and either diarrhea or constipation.

We need to make a key point that Hugh Trowell emphasized in the 1970s: it is important to look at fiber as a part of whole, unrefined foods. At times we have lost sight of the fact that the *fiber-rich foods are the ones delivering the greatest health benefits, and that you can't get all those benefits by extracting the fiber and just eating it by itself.* Antioxidants, polyunsaturated fatty acids, and phospholipids all have important effects on cell metabolism, as do the whole array of bioactive compounds, phytonutrients, vitamins, and minerals in high-fiber foods. So fiber-rich foods are very high in nutrients which have many beneficial dietary effects on the body.

Let me say something about *low carb*, which I am pleased to note is now phasing out. The pendulum swung much too far that way, allowing for an irrational faddishness, so it is a good thing that low-carb diets are now being discredited. They are unhealthy and not scientifically supported, and I consider those who pushed these high-fat, low-carb foods to be irresponsible.

I push plant-based foods. I think the diets around the world that have proved the healthiest for millennia are those that are highest in high-fiber foods. Invariably, those are plant-based foods and diets that use animal-meat products in moderation. Traditionally, the animals in these diets have been very low-fat range animals, wild animals, range-fed animals that are low in fat, or fish. A plant-based diet plus fish is, in my opinion, probably one of the healthiest diets we can promote. And I think if there is adequate calcium in a diet, a person could pretty much jettison the other animal products. Low-fat dairy, including skim milk, is a pretty good complement for some protein and for calcium, but I think it is possible to get by very well with a plant-based diet, adding some protein from soy foods that would negate the need for regular animal protein.

Antonia Trichopoulou, M.D.
Faculty of Medicine, University of Athens
Honorary President, Scientific Committee, Foundation for the Advancement
    of the Mediterranean Diet (Greece)
Editorial Board, Nutrition Journal
Director of the WHO Collaborating Centre of Nutrition, University
    of Athens

People in Greece consume a large amount of vegetables and legumes (beans), dress them with olive oil, add garlic and onions, and a lot of herbs, such as rosemary or oregano. We use hundreds of herbs in the Mediterranean cuisine—then at the end you have a very nice, tasty dish, which is not a side dish, it is not a salad, it's the main dish. Quite often in Greece when you ask people what they are going to eat for lunch or for dinner, they will tell you okra or beans or peas or eggplant. Traditionally, we don't eat a lot of meat (and when we do, the meat portions are not very big) and we eat fish once or twice a week.

A while ago, we decided to study and record some traditional Greek recipes, as we felt that in a few years nobody would be able to prepare them. We focused on the various greens used to prepare many traditional Greek green pies. There is a huge tradition for preparing pies with greens, and there are more than 100 greens to choose from. The old women know how to pick them from the mountains or the plains and understand how to combine them in order to prepare a tasty pie. We asked a lady to prepare a green pie with ten different greens for us (there are pies that have up to forty different greens), with additional garlic, onions, herbs, etc. My colleagues went to the mountains with her and picked over fifteen pounds of every green, and they also brought the whole pie into the laboratory. We lyophylized (freeze-dried) those greens and the full pie, and did chemical analysis for several antioxidants. There were many antioxidants and a surprising amount of quercetin (a polyphenol that is especially protective of capillary blood vessels). And of course the greens were a good source of fiber.

David Jenkins, M.D., Ph.D.
Professor, Department of Nutritional Sciences
University of Toronto and Saint Michael's Hospital

I think the ultimate diet would be what I am now calling eco-nutrition, and by that I mean something which is designed both for the planet and for the human genome. The program—rather than the diet because, in many ways, it's a way of life—would consist of exercise and calorie balance. It would not be about excess calories, but instead about a high-fiber, sometimes very high-fiber, diet, which would focus on a lot of leafy vegetables. In my opinion, leaves, with their fiber and their high antioxidant loads, have probably been neglected in the past, and they would be a very important part of the diet.

The protein foods, the nuts and the oil seeds, such as sesame seeds in their whole, unmodified form, should be a very important part of the program, both for the protein and for the oils. And then, of course, fruits in all their varieties should be included.

Finally, there are the cereals (grains), what I call my Neolithic extension (Neolithic referring to the cultural period beginning around 10,000 B.C. when agriculture began). I think it is important to have a variety of grains in the diet, and it is vital to have the grains as minimally extracted as possible because refining grains eliminates fiber, protein, and other nutrients.

PART THREE

Unveiling the Health Benefits of Whole-Plant Foods

17

What's with Fiber in Whole Grains?

The Wonders of a Grain Seed

As you drive on Highway 505 through the wheat fields of Northern California, the sign reads: "Farmers Feed America." It is a cry from the heart of people who know that their grain is a vital part of human food, as are the grains of barley, corn (maize), oats, rice, rye, sorghum, and teff. Grains are seeds. A complete new plant can grow from a seed, and that is why grains are such a rich nutrient source. A grain seed contains the parts of a complete new plant in the *germ,* and a generous supply of energy food in the starchy *endosperm,* the largest part of the grain. The *aleurone* layer surrounding the endosperm contains the B vitamins, and the minerals and enzymes that mobilize the starch, allowing its proper utilization in both plants and people. The entire grain is covered with a protective *bran* seed coat (*see* Figures 17.1 and 17.2) and protein is spread throughout the grain seed.

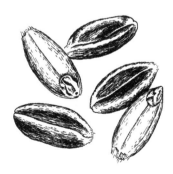

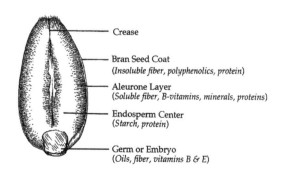

Crease

Bran Seed Coat
(*Insoluble fiber, polyphenolics, protein*)

Aleurone Layer
(*Soluble fiber, B-vitamins, minerals, proteins*)

Endosperm Center
(*Starch, protein*)

Germ or Embryo
(*Oils, fiber, vitamins B & E*)

Figure 17.1. Grain Seeds

Figure 17.2. Open Half Grain Seed

The Germ

The germ occupies only a small fraction of the grain seed, but the oils it provides are nutritionally very important, and include vitamin-E tocopherols, and phospholipids, the most common of which is lecithin. The essential oils in grain germ include the essential linolenic (omega-3) and linoleic (omega-6) fatty acids. The germ is also a rich source of folate, a B vitamin now considered even more important than previously thought. Low levels of folate in the diet are associated with a high incidence of spinal birth defects. Refined wheat flour is now enriched with folate, and even more folate is added to refined flour than would be found in the natural wheat germ, a compensatory effort by the millers to reduce the incidence of spinal birth defects. The presence of folate, or folic acid, also correlates well with low blood levels of homocysteine (a potentially toxic amino acid), which statistically correspond to reduced risk for many Western diseases, including Alzheimer's disease, cancer, diabetes, and heart disease.

The Seed Coat

A chaff, hull, husk, or shell usually covers seeds, but the seed coat itself is delicate enough to be eaten, especially after soaking or cooking. The protective outermost coatings of food seeds naturally soak up and hold water very well, in readiness for sprouting. In some cases, the seed coat imbibes water so well it becomes a gel. The bran seed coat of wheat will soak up water and simply expand because it is mostly insoluble fiber. In contrast, flaxseeds will form a soft gel when soaked in water, due to the presence of water-soluble fiber. Most seed coats of grains, including the underlying aleurone layer, are built from a mixture of soluble and insoluble fibers.

The seed coat provides more than physical protection and water-absorption capabilities, it also offers the seed protection against the aggressive effects of too much UV light from the sun and oxygen from the air. This is possible because, within the fiber matrix of the seed coat, there are antioxidant polyphenolic compounds that are also UV-light absorbers, to keep the rest of the seed from being affected by the UV light.

Phytic acid, or inositol hexaphosphate, is present in most seeds, in or near the seed coat where it holds valuable minerals ready for use by the growing plant. Inositol is a part of the vitamin B-complex and is released from the phytic acid, together with phosphate, when seeds are soaked or fermented. The enzyme phytase, which helps break down phytic acid, is also richly present in the seed coat. Soaking the grain releases the phytase for action, bringing about the decomposition of phytic acid and the release of minerals.

Because phytic acid can bind with mineral ions, it has been suspected of causing mineral deficiencies, but it has also been credited with anti-cancer effects, and this, along with its ability to supply inositol, phosphate, and minerals when suitably treated, suggests that phytic acid should be a welcome component of grains.

The Aleurone Layer

Very closely attached to the seed coat, between it and the endosperm, is the aleurone layer. Conveniently for the growing plant, the aleurone layer contains the B vitamins and minerals necessary for the release of energy from the carbohydrate food stored in the endosperm, and also for healthy cell multiplication.

The Endosperm

The large endosperm center in grains is primarily for storage of starch, and serves as an energy source for a new plant. The endosperm usually contains at least 10 percent protein, and the endosperm of some grains, such as oats, also contains a small amount of fat. Although the endosperm is a great source of energy foods in the form of digestible carbohydrates, it is almost devoid of B vitamins, minerals, protective polyphenolics, and fiber.

The Benefits of Whole Grains

Fiber and protective antioxidants are found particularly in the germ, the bran seed coat, and the aleurone layer, which surrounds the endosperm, immediately below the bran. There is relatively little fiber in the endosperm, so eating only the endosperm of grain seeds, as is the case with refined white wheat flour, means missing out on nutrients and fiber that are as essential for people as they are for the life of a new plant. Except for meat and mushrooms, only the seed foods (grains, legumes, and nuts) supply the B vitamins so well—all but vitamin B_{12}, which is not usually found in plant foods. Vegetarians cannot obtain enough vitamin B-complex unless they eat grain foods in their wholegrain form. The lack of B_{12} is a real drawback for vegans because this needed vitamin is primarily found in eggs, meat, milk, and milk products. There is some indication that seaweeds and fermented seed foods, such as miso and tempeh, contain vitamin B_{12}, but there still seems to be disagreement on whether the B_{12} from these sources is truly available.

The importance of whole grains in the diet, and their particular value in preventing and treating diabetes and coronary heart disease has been summarized by Dr. James Anderson:

"The specific benefits of wholegrain intake deserve special mention.

Whole grains appear to increase insulin sensitivity and reduce risk for developing diabetes and coronary heart disease. The bran layer of cereal grains is rich in fiber and phytochemicals that may have specific antioxidant, anti-inflammatory, phytoestrogen, and other effects that provide these benefits."

Weston Price was a dentist who traveled widely to see for himself the effects on bone structure and tooth decay of traditional diets that included whole grains versus refined-wheat diets. In 1939 he published a book, which showed graphically that people were born with better jaw bone structure if their parents ate grains in the whole form., and that eating refined flour and sugar caused tooth decay.

Breakfast Cereals of Today vs. Old-time Gruels and Porridges

Grains can be eaten raw. Have you ever seen farmers testing their wheat for harvest readiness? They crunch the wheat grains right there in the field, and if the grains are fully ripened, the gluten protein wads up just like chewing gum. A snack in bygone days was a pocketful of toasted rye or oats (grains taste better after they have been toasted, or if they are made into flour for bread or hot cereal). Whole grains have been central to the diet in most of the Western world since the beginnings of agriculture. The *porridges* and *gruels* of olden times were easy to make when grains were ground into a coarse or fine wholegrain flour. All that was needed was to add boiling water to the wholegrain flour, and stir well. When served as a sweet hot cereal, the grains were nevertheless mixed with a little salt, possibly some malt (the malt enzymes would make it sweet), and some fresh or cultured milk. Brown sugar, fruit, honey, or nuts were, and are still, options to add to the enjoyment. The ratio of water to wholegrain flour is 2 to 1 for a tasty, creamy-textured cereal. This was, and is, truly comfort food.

Words like *porridge* and *gruel* survive as food in children's stories (*Goldilocks and the Three Bears*), but have a very poor image in stories about grueling poverty and imprisonment. To escape this, and because they are now frequently made from commercially pretreated grains rather than wholegrain flours, the outdated words *porridge* or *gruel* have been replaced by the umbrella words *hot cereal,* in reference to both the commercial varieties and the organic wholegrain versions available at all health food stores and many upscale groceries. People are choosing the wholegrain organic cereals more and more, not just because they are more nutritious, but because they taste better.

When used in commercial hot cereals, wholegrain flours, flaked oats, and flaked barley cook faster than steel cut oats, which need more time for cooking. Today's commercial hot cereal is often pre-flavored with refined sugar and hydrogenated fat, both of which should be avoided for nutritional reasons, and if you wish to experience the full flavor and highly protective benefits of whole grains. When buying a hot cereal, it is important to read the label so you can avoid refined-grain products, refined sugars, hydrogenated fats, and trans fats. Similarly, cold cereals are often far from being wholegrain. They too can be replete with refined-grain products, added refined sugars, and hydrogenated and trans fats. If you value your health, such concoctions are to be avoided.

Almost all nutritionists agree that the healthiest way to eat grains is whole, with no parts removed, and preferably after a preparation method that releases the nutrients to a maximum. Examples include making hominy from corn, using enzyme-active malt in oatmeal, and making bread with enzyme-active malted grain and a sourdough starter.

The Whole Grains

Some of the grains, and the particular kinds of fiber and associated phytonutrients that each has to offer, are described below. The full nutritional benefits of these grains are only possible if the entire seed is eaten, without any processing or refinement that removes the nutrients. Common processing methods are mentioned for each of the plant foods described, and in terms of keeping the healthful parts of whole grains, some processing methods are better than others. In order to have the healthiest products, it is advisable to use the best from both the old and new methods for processing grain seeds. For good health, don't settle for eating less than the whole grain.

Amaranth

Among the indigenous crops of the ancient Incas, an amaranth seed known as kiwicha (*Amaranthus caudatus*) is perhaps the most nutritious of all grains because it has such a beneficial balance of amino acids in its protein, and an especially high lysine and tryptophan content. Along with starch and protein, there is a high proportion of fiber, due simply to its small size. The whole seed of amaranth is always eaten, whether it is puffed, ground into a flour, or eaten as a hot cereal. The full nutritional value of the whole seed that accompanies the fiber of amaranth is available—the B vitamins, germ oils, insoluble fiber, minerals, phytonutrients that include antioxidant polyphenolics, and vitamin E.

Amaranth was abandoned as a crop after the Spanish conquest, and it was only revived in the late 1900s. Amaranth is wonderfully drought-tolerant and therefore has great value as a dependable crop in areas where few other crops can survive, regardless of any climate shift, from year to year. The renewed popularity of kiwicha amaranth has been so great that it is now widely available.

In Latin America, amaranth is either boiled for hot cereal, puffed, or made into flour for tortillas. In North America the grain is used the same way, including for amaranth tortillas, which are delicious, and in the Himalayas, where other varieties are grown, amaranth is also ground into flour and made into unleavened flat breads. Amaranth starch is unusually gooey in texture after cooking and is similar to the starch found in sticky, glutinous rice.

Barley

Barley and wheat are the most ancient of the cultivated grains, but perhaps the only remaining frequent home use for barley in North America is as pearled barley in soups. Barley is available in health food stores, and it is still used in pancake mixes and as a hot cereal by a few health-conscious Americans. Breads are made from barley in several countries, including Ethiopia, Finland, the Middle East, Scotland, and Tibet. Substantial amounts of barley are made into malt and used for making beer. Various concentrated extracts of roasted barley malt are used to give color, flavor, sweetness, and added nutritional value to all kinds of processed foods, including coffee alternatives, chocolate, and soft drinks. Small amounts of barley malt flour are widely used as an additive to wheat flour in breadmaking.

The barley of the ancients was the free-threshing type, known today as hull-less barley. When hull-less barley is harvested, the grain is easily freed from the husk or hull, leaving the bran seed coat intact. A more common type of barley available today has the husk attached to the bran seed coat so it cannot be easily removed from the barley seeds, which is appropriate for making malt extracts and beer.

Pearled barley for soup has the husk removed by abrasion in a suitably designed stone mill. The extent of the pearling process is variable. Minimal pearling would only remove the husk and outermost bran layer, but further abrasion could remove all of the germ and the aleurone layer. This results in overly pearled barley that lacks bran fiber with its associated polyphenolic antioxidants, and also lacks the beneficial oils of the germ and the B vitamins associated with the aleurone layer. Barley flakes are also available as an alternative to oat flakes for cooked cereal, but if they are made with pearled barley they are unlikely to be as nutritionally valuable as oat flakes from whole oats.

Barley endosperm contains the expected carbohydrate and protein energy store, and also a small amount of lipids. Starch is the most abundant carbohydrate in the endosperm, but as in oats there is a substantial amount of soluble dietary fiber carbohydrate present in the form of beta-glucan. Beta-glucan is gummy in texture when plenty of water is present and it gives pearled barley its characteristic texture when cooked. This type of soluble fiber is valuable because it promotes the growth of beneficial bacteria in the colon.

Hull-less barley, in a wholegrain form as a soup or cereal, or as whole barley flour in breads is a better choice than pearled barley. Hull-less barley will supply all the wholegrain fiber—the insoluble fiber from the bran, the soluble fiber from the endosperm, and still more fiber from the germ. Associated with all this fiber will be the vitamin-E tocopherols and oils from the germ, and the B vitamins and minerals in the aleurone layer around the endosperm. Barley is beneficial for preventing arteriosclerosis, and the phytonutrients present, including the antioxidant polyphenolics in the bran, are contributing their effect in conjunction with the beta-glucan from the endosperm.

The traditional Scottish bannock bread made from barley also contains buttermilk, and its acidity greatly aids the release of minerals held by the phytic acid in the aleurone layer. An ancient way of preparing barley flour was to first toast the grain, probably to dry it sufficiently to ensure storage that was free from insect or fungal damage. This toasted grain makes a most delicious flour to use for bannocks or scones. Authors Jeffrey Alford and Naomi Duguid (*Flatbreads and Flavors*) found exactly this kind of flour eaten as a cereal with tea in Tibet.

Barley Malt. The first stage in the malting process is to sprout the grain. The simplest malt is just gently dried, sprouted grain, and it retains all its enzyme activity. More complex malts are roasted to varying degrees, and the remaining enzyme activity varies accordingly. The presence of the attached barley husk protects the embryonic plant when piles of the sprouting barley are raked to promote even exposure to the air. The husk also acts as a filter. The liquid that is fermented to make beer, is produced by soaking coarsely ground malt in hot water. During this process, known as *mashing,* the temperature is generally maintained at 60–70°C (140–158°F). At this temperature, the starch is gelatinized and can be rapidly broken down into soluble sugars by the enzyme alpha-amylase. Several enzymes, including phytase, are also active at this temperature, and they release other soluble substances from the barley, such as B vitamins, minerals, oligosaccharides (soluble-fiber carbohydrates), and polyphenolics. Less heat-tolerant enzymes are deactivated. At the end of the mash, the liquid containing all the soluble substances from the barley is filtered through the husks that sink to the bottom of the vat, and drained off. This liquid product is known as malt extract, the same malt extract that is concentrated into a syrup, and is available in jars or cans (the heat needed to concentrate the malt extract to a syrup destroys the enzyme activity). Home beermakers are familiar with a variety of malt extract syrups, to which they add water and proceed to ferment into beer. Syrups of barley-malt extract are deliciously flavored and sweet, as well as being enormously nutritious. During World War II, children in Britain, myself included, gladly ate barley malt extract by the tablespoonful. Eating the barley malt syrup was my introduction to its gooeyness, sweetness, and good-for-you qualities. We also ate a deliciously gooey malt bread at tea time that was made by adding raisins and a syrup of barley malt extract for flavor and texture. Also, I always visited my grandparents in northeast England for the summer, and the walk into town took us past the magnificent aroma of roasting barley issuing forth from a malting factory.

During the early stages of roasting sprouted barley grains, the enzyme action results in sugars and flavor compounds, such as polyphenolics, being released, just as in the mashing process. When the temperature is further raised, the enzymes break down and the barley dries out. The final *malted barley* can range in color from pale tan to dark brown. All barley malts are much more flavorful than the barley from which they are produced.

Barley malt flour is used in breads, as an often unnoticed flour additive that supplies needed enzymes. For this, the barley sprouts are not roasted, but are dried at warm room temperature, which preserves most of all the increased B vitamins and enzymes resulting from the sprouting. The husk is removed by abrasion, or pearling, and an enzyme-active barley malt flour is produced by milling the sprouted seed. Vitamin and enzyme content will be highest if the whole seed, including the bran and sprout, is present in the final barley malt flour. Wheat and rye are also used similarly to produce an enzyme-active malt flour, but barley malt flour is the most commonly made and is easily obtained for breadmaking.

The nutritional value of barley is greatly enhanced by sprouting. Common barley with its attached husk is the type that is generally sprouted for the various types of malt, and it is steeped in water as the first step in the process. During the steeping, or soaking, the husk, bran, and aleurone layer release soluble materials that can be carried into the barley endosperm. Some of the most important solubles carried into the endosperm are polyphenolics from the husk and the bran, B vitamins and enzymes from the aleurone layer, and minerals released from the aleurone layer. This has very important consequences for the nutritional value of barley malt because, when it is dried and pearled, many of the phenolics, B vitamins, and enzymes associated with the outermost layer are retained in the barley malt. Even when the bran is removed in a roller-milling process, barley malt flour can still contain a rich concentration of nutrients. Barley malt extracts are rich in soluble fiber in the form of gummy beta-glucans. They are sweet with malt sugar derived from the starch by the enzymes. Their color results from the sugar caramelization during the roasting process, and their flavor and aroma come largely from the phenolic compounds.

Buckwheat

One of the daily pleasures of living here in the United States is the possibility of meeting people from every corner of this planet, and also sampling much of their food. Invitingly packaged among the mounds of Italian-style pasta in upscale grocery stores are Japanese soba noodles made entirely from buckwheat flour. East European buckwheat kasha can be found among the cereals, and buckwheat flour for blini pancakes can be found with the flours.

Buckwheat (*Fagopyrum esculentum*) is a very hardy plant in the same family as sorrel and rhubarb. Since it is completely unrelated to wheat, buckwheat is a suitable food for anyone who is allergic to wheat gluten. In cross section, the buckwheat seed is distinctively triangular. When the husk is cracked open, it can be winnowed away, leaving the seed with a thin bran and germ intact; this is the wholegrain buckwheat groat, called kasha when it is roasted. Ground into a flour, kasha is the basis for a simple hot cereal made by adding boiling water, salt if you wish, and stirring. With various accompaniments it can be served at every meal. Buckwheat blini pancakes are usually yeast-leavened, but historically they must have been naturally fermented with a more complex culture that probably included lactic bacteria. Whole buckwheat groats can be cooked the same way as rice.

The buckwheat plant is rich in rutin, which was among the first of the antioxidant bioflavonoids (colored polyphenolics) to be recognized. Back in the 1930s, researcher Albert Szent-Györgyi and his co-workers tried hard to gain vitamin status for these bioflavonoids. Now, seventy years later, the benefits of this type of compound are at last being appreciated, regardless of their status as a vitamin or not. The benefits of rutin, such as the protection of capillary blood vessels and the enhancement of the effects of vitamin C, were all reported back in the 1930s by Dr. Szent-Györgyi.

In Tibet, the leaves of a perennial buckwheat are eaten as a salad, and they provide a rich source of the beneficial rutin. These and similar foods explain the hardiness of the Tibetan mountain people who are compelled to live on plants, such as buckwheat, that can survive the severe climate.

Fortunately, all parts of the buckwheat seed are usually included in buckwheat flour—bran, germ, and endosperm. Antioxidant polyphenolics, including rutin, are particularly associated with the insoluble bran fiber and the germ, as are the B vitamins, especially niacin and vitamin B_6. The total fiber in buckwheat groats is 10 percent, including 9 percent insoluble fiber. In the search for drugs to treat diabetes, buckwheat extract has recently demonstrated some success.

Corn

Growing up in Britain, I certainly knew cornflakes for breakfast, and saw that those girls aspiring to be film stars in Hollywood made certain they had cornflakes as part of their breakfast. Actually, American corn is known as maize in Britain and most other countries; British corn is wheat, and we also had wheat flakes. At that time, I was less in tune with the distinction, except that wheat flakes seemed to be more sustaining. In fact, wheat flakes are usually made from whole wheat, whereas cornflakes are made only from the endosperm of the corn seed. Fortunately, cornflakes are flavored with barley malt, which supplies a few B vitamins and a little soluble fiber to supplement the small amount of resistant corn starch in cornflakes. Ironically, Dr. J. H. Kellogg's idea was to make whole-kernel cornflakes, which he did successfully. But his cornflakes made with wholegrain corn rapidly turned rancid, due to the presence of corn oil that is easily oxidized once it is released from the intact corn. It was not until 1903 that his brother, W. K. Kellogg, found a way to degerminate the corn before making the cornflakes. Since then, Kellogg's cornflakes have been made with degerminated corn and consequently lack the nutrients associated with the germ, such as vitamins B and E. Most breakfast cereals now, including cornflakes, are enriched by adding B vitamins and minerals to partially compensate for this deficiency, but there is no compensation for the fiber that is removed.

Ancient uses for corn as a staple involved wholegrain corn, but many versions today are devoid of corn germ, bran, and the aleurone layer. Thin flat breads, cereals, and roasted cornmeal are the most significant of the original corn foods. Corn is the most widely grown of any cereal crop, and each country has its own characteristic ways of enjoying it. Perhaps the most popular corn foods in North America other than corn-on-the-cob, cornflakes, and popcorn, are tortillas and corn chips of Mexican origin, polenta from Italy, and pinole meal of Mexican and American Hopi Indian origin. Pinole is roasted, ground wholegrain corn made into a delicious breakfast beverage with water and milk, and flavored with cinnamon and brown sugar. When corn is eaten as a staple, especially by the poor, it is particularly important for it to be as nutritious as possible. The Mexicans know how to obtain the greatest food value from wholegrain corn. They first make it into nixtamal, using a very ancient process of cooking it in water made alkaline with wood ash or lime, and then allowing the corn to soak in the alkaline water as it cools. To make tortillas, the drained nixtamal is washed free of some of the thin hull, drained, and then ground to a doughy mass on a grinding stone before being shaped into thin tortillas or tortilla chips and baked on a griddle. The preparation of hominy is similar to nixtamal, and the method was taught to early settlers by Native Americans. Dried nixtamal can be stored easily and is much less vulnerable to insect or mold damage than untreated whole corn. Ground dried nixtamal is generally known as masa flour and is also much more stable than whole cornmeal—the germ oils, particularly, are stabilized in the nixta-

Pellagra

Corn is also deficient in the amino acid tryptophan, a precursor for nicotinic acid and the related niacin. Poor people all over the world who subsist on corn are vulnerable to the niacin-deficiency disease pellagra unless they have treated their corn with alkaline water to render the niacin available for digestion. The pellagra symptoms are often described as the three D's: dementia, dermatitis (manifested by an extreme sensitivity to sunlight), and diarrhea. Italian polenta corn is not treated with alkali before milling, and poor Italians were plagued with pellagra in much the same way as poor Americans living in the South who did not make their corn into hominy. Enrichment of refined cornmeal with vitamins, including niacin, and general improvement in the availability of a variety of foods, especially milk, has led to a gradual disappearance of pellagra. It is now seen only occasionally around the world, except for southern Africa where there are still many cases.

Pellagra was unknown in the classical Western world. In Spain, it was first noticed in 1735 after the introduction of corn from the Americas into Europe, and in Italy in 1771. In North America, pellagra was a significant disease from just after the Civil War in the late 1860s until the United States began enriching refined flours with B vitamins, including niacin, in the 1940s.

mal and do not turn rancid so easily. The treatment with the alkaline water separates the layers of fiber that form the thin hull on the corn seed, and this is usually rubbed off before the corn is wet-milled into a dough before being shaped. Below the hull is, first, a thin bran seed coat layer and then the aleurone layer. Provided the nixtamal has not been milled to cause loss of the germ, bran, and aleurone layers, the resulting cornmeal will be rich in B vitamins, minerals, carotenoid pigments, which are vitamin A precursors in yellow-corn varieties, tocopherols, and linoleic (omega-6) acid, one of the essential fatty acids. Presumably the B vitamins can migrate from the aleurone layer into the endosperm of the corn during the soaking of corn to make nixtamal. Niacin in particular becomes much more readily available as a result of making corn into nixtamal. Other grains, such as wheat, actually have a lower niacin content, but in those it is more readily absorbed during digestion.

Today, a great deal of the corn intended for human use is untreated with alkali and is degerminated and debranned during milling into corn grits. Most corn grits are essentially endosperm and are devoid of fiber and the associated aleurone layer and B vitamins. Breakfast cornflakes, and the various corn puffs and balls are generally made from these grits and are not only devoid of the nutritional benefits of the bran germ and aleurone layer, but are also relatively low in protein—corn endosperm is much lower in protein than wheat or rice endosperm. Refined corn products are among the highest starch foods available, and can contribute significant extra calories when eaten as snack foods. True popcorn is usually made by heating a particular type of flinty corn, which is whole kernel and will deliver the beta-carotenes, B vitamins, corn germ oil, minerals, and tocopherols associated with the germ and bran fiber of the corn seed coat. All these nutrients will balance and improve the assimilation of the starch from the endosperm in a way that is missing from the refined corn snacks and cereals, unless they have been suitably fortified with B vitamins. Even then, the fortification does not replace all the nutrients removed during the milling of the corn into grits.

Corn-based foods made from lime-treated corn are usually wholegrain foods, and provide the B vitamins, minerals, and germ oils closely associated with the fibrous bran. In general, only the thin hull that could supply even more fiber is missing. Many of these whole kernel foods are fried, and it is important to avoid anything processed with hydrogenated fats, or excessive amounts of any fat, even the healthiest type. Tortilla chips are most commonly produced by frying, although there are some excellent baked tortilla chips, notably blue corn chips, which are widely sold. Soft, whole corn tortillas and hominy are perhaps the healthiest of all the corn-based foods.

Millet

Millet is rarely eaten in North America, but it is a delicately flavored grain that is favored as an alternative to wheat for those allergic to wheat gluten. Millet makes a very pleasing hot cereal and can be an alternative to rice as a dinner grain. Millet is also added to multigrain breads.

The difficulty with millet is knowing which kind to describe. The word *millet* is applied broadly to a variety of millets, including pearl, and even to teff, an entirely different grain (in this context, the word *pearl* refers to the type of millet, not its processing). Millet is a valuable crop in Africa because it can be grown under conditions that would not support crops, such as wheat, rice, corn (maize), or barley, so it helps reduce the risk of famine.

Pearl millet is the type most often sold in North America, and as a whole grain it supplies the vitamins and minerals associated with the germ and fibrous seed coat, especially folic acid, potassium, and thiamine. The fiber in the seed coat is mostly insoluble fiber (80 percent of the total fiber), with a small but significant amount of soluble fiber. Millet contributes only about two-thirds the fiber that the same weight of whole wheat can contribute to the diet.

Oats

Oats are the traditional grain of the Scots and Irish, eaten mostly as hot cereal, which they call porridge, and a variety of oatcakes. So it was astonishing to drive in Scotland during the 1980s and not be able to buy the old-fashioned porridge for breakfast at several restaurants I visited, ones which nevertheless always served white toast. Oatmeal is much more available in the United States, and has a deservedly good reputation as a healthy wholegrain cereal. In a recent study on children and teenagers, those who regularly ate oatmeal for breakfast were 50 percent less likely to become overweight. This was attributed to their higher fiber intake as a result of eating oatmeal. Which brings me to the real meaning of the word *oatmeal*—it is oats ground to a meal in a mill. Originally it was this oatmeal that was made into a hot cereal. This practice was so common that the hot cereal itself is still referred to as oatmeal, but today's oat milling generally produces rolled oats or oat flakes, which are made into a hot cereal.

The husk of oats is strongly attached, so after harvesting and cleaning, it must be removed with an oat-hulling machine. The whole oat seed freed from the husk is the groat. Stone mills fell out of use for all the grains, including oats, in the late 1800s. Many stone mills were highly specialized and various steel mills were invented to do the tasks once achieved with stone mills, including the dehusking of oats. The steel mills invented for cutting groats in 1875 produced coarsely cut pieces, steel-cut oats, instead of the fluffy and somewhat flaky textured oatmeal previously produced by stone mills for millennia. The disadvantage of steel-cut oats is that they take longer to cook than the stone-milled oatmeal, which was almost instantly cooked by adding boiling water. As can be imagined, oatmeal from the less popular steel-cut oats became rare by the beginning of the 1900s and was replaced by quicker cooking rolled oats. The solution was to partially steam the groats or steel-cut oats, then pass them through steel rollers, which turned them into the flakes now called oatmeal or baby oats.

Today, oat flour is produced from steamed groats that are milled to a flour by one of several methods, such as hammer milling or roller milling. Roller milling is generally used to produce a refined endosperm flour. Stone milling is still used occasionally, but most likely with stones that are not particularly prepared for oats. Steaming, which is part of the flaking process, is advantageous in preserving the processed oats against rancidity. This is because the enzymes that would cause degradation when brought into action by moistening the oats are inactivated by the heat of the steam. The care that was once taken to use really fresh oat flour is rare now. Instead of storing the oat flour, the clean groats were stored in a covered wooden box in a dry area, and milled only as needed, and the flour produced this way was probably used up in a month or two. The two main uses for fresh oat flour in the old days were for porridge and oatcakes, the latter made from a stiff oatmeal porridge dough flattened to a thin disk and then baked on a griddle. Today's oat flour is used for baby food and ready-to-eat cereals, and is seldom sold as oat flour.

Wholegrain oats have somehow survived almost completely intact through all the possible methods for refining it that are available today (exceptions are separated oat fractions, such as oat bran and refined oat flour, which cannot be regarded as wholegrain products). Oat endosperm is mostly made up from starch and beta-glucan, some lipids, and protein of a higher quality than in wheat. The protein quality is especially good because it contains a relatively high proportion of lysine that allows good protein assimilation (lysine is usually found in much lower proportion in other cereals). Of greatest interest here is the beta-glucan, which is a soluble fiber with cholesterol-lowering properties. It is the gummy beta-glucan that gives oatmeal its characteristic texture. Both starch and beta-glucan are built up from glucose units, but with different linkages that cause a change in properties. Beta-glucan is a dietary fiber gum, which is not digested until it reaches the bacterial enzymes of the colon. Short-chain fatty acids produced in the colon by the bacterial action are absorbed and cause a favorable cholesterol profile in the blood. This beta-glucan is distributed most richly around the outside of the oat endosperm, just under the aleurone layer. So we have an explanation for the popularity of oat bran to lower cholesterol, provided that the bran is separated together with the outer layer of the endosperm.

The oat germ is exceptionally rich in oils and oily textured substances, all of which are valuable for good health. Oat oil has a high content of more-unsaturated oleic and linoleic (omega-6) acids, and a polyunsaturated-to-saturated fatty acid ratio of 2.2 to 1, well above the recommended ratio of at least 1 to 1. Included in oat oil are sterols and sterol esters that can lower cholesterol, phospholipids that are related to lecithin, and vitamin-E tocopherols that are powerful antioxidants and contribute to the good health of the cardiovascular and reproductive systems.

The phenolic antioxidants are well represented in the oat bran fiber and have even been extracted for use as a natural antioxidant preservative for other foods. The importance of the many phenolic and polyphenolic compounds found in plant foods has not yet been fully explored. For oats this is particularly relevant because the healthy effects of eating whole oats seem greater than can be explained by considering only the currently described nutrients found in oats, such as beta-glucans and antioxidant lipids.

Oat fiber is usually eaten as a part of the whole oat grain and is well-accompanied by major nutrients and protective compounds. In whole oats, the B vitamins and minerals are also well represented.

The reduction of phytic acid in oats results from moistening processes and fermentations, including the addition of cultured milk. In the past, all these processes were used for the various oat dishes that were prepared in Scotland. It is likely that the addition of water before steaming oats also begins the conversion of phytic acid to inositol, part of the vitamin B-complex. With all their benefits, oats deserve an even greater popularity as part of a healthy diet than they enjoy at the moment.

Quinoa

Quinoa (pronounced *keen-wah*) is one of the three ancient high-altitude grains of the Incas: kaniwa (*Chenopodium pallidicaule*), kiwicha (*Amaranthus caudatus*) and quinoa (*Chenopodium quinoa*). Although some of the quinoa grown in the Andes is exported, most of it in North America probably comes from Canada and Colorado. Quinoa that is imported from Bolivia and Peru is grown and harvested just as it was hundreds of years ago, with all the work done manually by the local villagers. The plants are threshed by bashing bunches of them on the ground. After allowing the wind to winnow away the husks, the quinoa grains are washed and dried.

Quinoa is a delicious alternative to rice, and is similarly boiled in water, but for a much shorter time. Nutritionally, quinoa is a superior grain because it has such a lot of high-quality protein (16–23 percent), with high levels of the essential amino acids cystine, lysine, and methionine (the high level of lysine complements other grains, such as corn). Another remarkable feature of quinoa is the large germ, or embryo, that can be as much as 60 percent of the seed—this gives the seed a 4–9-percent fat content that is rich in linoleic (omega-6) acid. You can see the embryo clearly, wound all around the endosperm, especially after cooking. The pleasing starchiness of the endosperm is evident in the eating.

The quinoa seed coat has a delicate powdery structure and is rich in saponins, so-called because they foam like soap in water. Saponins are also bitter in flavor and were historically removed by soaking, washing, and rubbing the seeds in water. The quinoa currently available in North America has a pleasant, mild flavor reminiscent of sesame, and most of the saponins have usually been washed away. Removing the saponins this way leaves the vitamin content of the seed basically untouched—the seed is still viable and can be sprouted even after this washing. In the plant, the saponins are necessary to protect it from birds and insects, and research has now found that they lower cholesterol very effectively by binding with it, so any small amount of saponins that remains after washing the quinoa seeds is therefore beneficial.

Quinoa seeds have a distinctly different shape from wheat or rye seeds. Instead of a bran coat, there is a powdery layer of saponins. The fibrous part of the quinoa seed is the embryo that winds all around the seed and becomes highly visible after cooking. It contains mostly insoluble fiber (86 percent of the total fiber) that contributes very few calories. Quinoa contributes less than half the amount of fiber of whole wheat, but its fiber is intertwined with all the components of the embryo plant, especially the B vitamins and the oils that are rich in linoleic (omega-6) acid.

Rice

When brown rice was finally polished to the bright white of rice eaters' dreams, the serious disease beriberi instantly became rampant among poor rice-eating people in almost every region in the rice-eating world. Beriberi results from a deficiency of thiamine, which is vitamin B_1, and is found in health-giving quantity in the aleurone layer of the rice grain. Dry beriberi has symptoms related to nerve damage that causes paralysis and muscle wasting.

Wet beriberi causes edema and heart failure. This damage arises because thiamine is needed to utilize carbohydrates, and the process of polishing rice white removes the aleurone layer and the thiamine, causing a deficiency. Babies can also become sick and die suddenly if their mothers' milk does not supply adequate amounts of thiamine.

Milling methods for practically all grains were changed in the late 1800s when milling engineers thought they could invent machines that would achieve whatever was wanted. In the case of rice, people thought that by removing all the germ, all the brown bran, and all the underlying brown aleurone layer, they would have the perfect white-colored rice grain. This dream turned into the nightmare of thiamine deficiency and the resulting disease beriberi. For some, it is alleviated by spraying thiamine and other B vitamins back onto the white rice. Rice with thiamine sprayed on should ideally not be washed, or only minimally washed, before cooking, to avoid losing the B vitamins again. Cooking the rice so all the water is absorbed will conserve all the nutrients associated with the rice grain, no matter how it has been processed. This is the preferred method for good nutrition, just as the preferred form for good nutrition is whole brown rice. Predictably, whiteness in grains became distinctly unattractive once we realized what we were missing in the brown-colored bran and germ—white rice is something we avoid just as strongly as white pasta and white bread.

Although beriberi rampaged when white rice became the rice of choice, mysteriously, most people on the Indian continent seemed immune to it. This mystery—why much of India avoided beriberi even though they also polished their rice—was one of the first to be solved at the beginning of nutrition science and resulted in the discovery of thiamine.

In the early 1900s, Malaya became home for immigrants from China and Tamil (in southern India), who all ate polished white rice as their staple food. By this time, beriberi had become epidemic, with its cause still unknown, so Dr. W. L. Braddon, who was in Malaya around 1907, was amazed to see that beriberi seemed to strike the Chinese population, but the people from Tamil seemed unaffected. In studying the diets of the each group, he found that the only difference in their food was how they processed their rice *before* polishing it. The Chinese ate milled, polished white rice and the Tamil Indians parboiled their rice before polishing it.

Building on this preliminary evidence that parboiled rice could cure and prevent beriberi, Dr. William Fletcher proceeded to supervise feeding parboiled white rice to the inmates of a mental asylum in Kuala Lumpur, the capital of Malaya. As a result of his efforts, beriberi was almost completely eliminated in the asylum, and many examples of beriberi being eradicated by eating parboiled white rice followed. But, of course, there was another way the disease could be eliminated—by eating *un*polished brown rice, an observation made Dr. Edward Vedder in 1909 when he advised local Philippine scouts under American army officers to change their rations from polished white rice to a mixture of dried beans and unpolished brown rice. Eventually the compound thiamine was isolated from parboiled white rice and was used alone to cure beriberi, but this was not until 1932. (*See* the inset on page 95 for an explanation of how the thiamine arrives in the endosperm of parboiled rice.)

When rice is harvested with a combine harvester today, the grains are still in their husks and the product is known as paddy, or rough rice. Removal of the rice husk from paddy is not easy, but ancient people nevertheless achieved it using two primary methods: either pounding rough rice with a wooden pestle in a deep stone mortar to break off the husk, or parboiling the rough rice to swell the kernel sufficiently to burst open the husk and release it after drying. Pounding cracked the husk and released the rice kernel with practically all the bran and germ intact. Winnowing the husks away was another necessary step achieved by hand, and brown rice, complete with all the bran and germ, was the final product. The method is physically demanding, so it is not surprising that a small machine, the Engelberg rice mill, became enormously popular—it husked the rice, polished the rice with an abrasive steel roller, and fanned or sieved away the unwanted husk and polishings of bran and germ, all in a single pass. But it was invented prior to discovering that the bran and germ of grains were so incredibly valuable for our health. Before the Engelberg machine was invented, sophisticated stone mills were used for husking rice in America. Oliver Evans, from Delaware, who wrote *The Young Mill-Wright and Miller's Guide*, a definitive book about stone milling in 1795, includes a description of a stone mill designed to husk rice. The stones are picked full of large holes, and are set more than the length of the grain apart. In principle, the rough rice husks are forcibly rubbed against each other and they husk themselves. Rice-husking stones were used elsewhere, including China, where the stones can still be found in museum displays. In his description, Evans makes no mention of attempting to polish the rice, and beriberi was unknown in his lifetime (he died in 1819). Unfortunately, the art of preparing these stone mills became lost in favor of today's steel-husking machines, some of which actually have a design reminiscent of a stone mill.

Is there a connection between the longevity of the Japanese and their predilection for brown rice? The oldest Japanese man recently died in his sleep, at the age of 114 years, and there is a Japanese woman still living who is now 114 years old. Both are from the most southern island in Japan, far from crowded Tokyo, and have most likely eaten brown rice their entire life. Although many Japanese like to store their rice as whole-kernel brown rice, and polish it just before using, there are still a substantial number of Japanese in the countryside who actually eat their rice brown. According to a 1983 article, restaurants serving brown rice are on the increase in both the cities and the countryside in Japan. Brown rice stays sweet-flavored and is highly suitable for long-term storage. That is quite a thought, considering how much effort is made to stabilize the bran removed from rice as nutrient-rich polishings for animal feed. The instability of the rice polishings is due to the release of enzymes from ruptured cells of the aleurone layer, bran, and germ. Some of these enzymes can break down the oils and allow them to be oxidized,

Parboiled Rice

The distribution of nutrients in parboiled, or converted rice, as it is sometimes called, differs from brown rice prepared by dry milling processes. Parboiling rice as a method for husking rough rice causes the nutrients in the bran and germ to be drawn into the endosperm. During the soaking step for parboiled rice, water gradually penetrates the outside husk, the bran, and finally the endosperm, carrying with it the B vitamins thiamine and niacin, and antioxidant phenolics. There are many methods for parboiling rice, but the essential steps are to first soak the rough rice in hot water for a few hours, then drain off excess water, steam the rice, and finally dry it. The effect of this processing is to gelatinize the starch in the endosperm and harden the rice grain, as well as burst open the husk so it is easily removed.

Parboiling is an ancient method that makes it easier to remove the husks when using either primitive pounding methods or modern steel-milling equipment. Parboiled brown rice has fewer nutrients than plainly milled brown rice, but it is still better to eat parboiled rice in the brown form because only a portion of the nutrients pass into the endosperm during parboiling. The remainder of the B vitamins, the insoluble fiber, the minerals, and the germ oils are all present in the outside layers of brown parboiled rice.

Puffed rice cereals and puffed rice cakes are made from precooked or parboiled rice. Both are tastier and more nutritious when they are made from brown rice.

causing rancidity. The solution is usually to heat the rice polishings, or rice bran, to inactivate the enzymes. The intact grain of carefully hulled brown rice has a full quota of antioxidants that prevent the oils from turning rancid, especially while they are contained in their original cells. These are the same antioxidants that protect against arteriosclerosis and give a healthy cholesterol profile. All these antioxidants are associated with the fiber in the aleurone layer, bran, and germ of brown rice, and include generous amounts of phenolics and vitamin-E tocopherols. The B vitamins, especially thiamine and niacin, are distributed between the bran and germ (unless the rice has been parboiled, there is very little in the endosperm), and valuable amounts of minerals are also associated with the rice bran and aleurone layer. White rice, which consists only of endosperm, is therefore naturally lacking adequate amounts of these essential vitamins. Rice-bran fiber is mostly composed of insoluble fiber, and has only trace amounts of soluble fiber.

Rye

Rye is the grain used to make the intriguing black breads of Scandinavia and Eastern Europe. Danish dark rye sliced thinly for open sandwiches, German pumpernickel and Russian borodinski from rye and wheat, flavored with caraway and coriander, are just the beginning of a long list of delicious rye breads. Cookbook recipes often include darkening agents, but the original way to produce a black bread was to use whole grains and a sourdough, and bake it at the temperature of boiling water for a long time. To achieve the right conditions in Iceland, they use the natural steam that comes up through holes in the lava-flow landscape. In *The Great Scandinavian Baking Book*, author Beatrice Ojakangas describes how this steam is also used to heat Icelandic homes, greenhouses, and cattle barns as well as steam ovens. Icelandic dark rye, baked at steam temperature, is left to bake for many hours in a closed pan, and under these conditions, the bread darkens and develops an amazing sweetness and chocolate aroma.

Another part of rye's appeal is the spongy, gummy texture of the breads, similar to that of oats and barley. In rye, this gumminess is due to pentosans, which, like glucans, are not digested until they reach the microorganisms of the colon, which classifies them as soluble fiber. Oat and barley glucans are built from glucose units, and rye pentosans are built from pentose sugars, such as arabinose and xylose. The properties of rye's pentosan gum are similar to glucan gum. Pentosans enhance the way in which the rye dough will hold water (bakers will understand this). Rye bread texture therefore benefits from *whole* rye flour that naturally contains the highest amounts of soluble pentosan gum. Rye is a soft grain, and stone-milling whole rye for bread-making does not produce enough damaged starch for optimal water-holding ability. Rye bread texture and flavor also benefit by making a mash from a portion of the whole rye flour, malt, and hot water. Making a mash at 60–70°C (140–158°F) for one to three hours, gelatinizes the starch and speeds up the action of enzymes, such as alpha-amylase and phytase, while deactivating others, such as beta-amylase. In addition, the gelatinized starch enhances the water-holding capacity of rye doughs. The lightest rye breads are made when enough water is used to fully hydrate the bran and still give a self-supporting dough. Stone-milling rye to a fine-textured wholegrain flour is easy, provided the rye is sufficiently dry. Fortunately from the point of view of good health, rye is quite difficult to successfully roller-mill to a refined endosperm flour, mostly because the pentosans produce a gumminess during the initial moisturizing, or tempering, of the grain.

Scandinavian Whole Rye Breads. Scandinavians who consistently eat whole rye breads seem to have an advantage over those who eat refined wheat and rye breads. This in part helps to explain why, in 1978, colon cancer rates were found to be much lower in the small Finnish village of Kuopio than in Copenhagen, Denmark. Both places have similar Scandinavian-style food, but the Kuopio rye bread is made from wholegrain flour, and very little refined rye or wheat bread is eaten. In Copenhagen, refined wheat- and rye-flour breads are readily available. In Kuopio the insoluble rye-bran fiber, along with the antioxidant polyphenolics in the rye bran, were helping to protect against colon cancer.

Coarsely ground whole rye is used for the denser rye breads. With wheat, there is a clear correlation between the volume of a loaf from whole grain and the fineness of the flour. The finer the flour, the larger the volume of the loaf; it's all about the availability of the starch and protein to form the bread texture. There are also differences in the effects of eating coarse whole-rye breads as opposed to fine whole-rye breads. The digestible starch, the protein, and the fats in whole rye are less available from coarse flour than from fine flour. Bread made from a coarse flour will have more starch that resists digestion before reaching the colon than bread from a fine flour, which can be digested and absorbed within an hour or less. The resistant starch acts like soluble dietary fiber and will not be an energy source until several hours later, when it has been broken down and absorbed following bacterial action in the colon. Even then the pathway is different. Whereas digested starch is absorbed as glucose, the resistant starch is degraded to, and absorbed as, short-chain fatty acids, the same acids found in sourdough bread as a result of lactic fermentation. Acetic, propionic and butyric acids are the most common short-chain fatty acids produced, along with lactic acid.

The advantage of glucose being released into the blood slowly is that the glucose can usually be used steadily until the next meal. The blood can only hold a small amount of glucose before it is stored as glycogen or fat as a result of the natural effect of insulin. So if the glucose can be used as energy at the same speed that it is entering the blood, there will be less probability of it being converted to fat by a large insulin surge. When short-chain fatty acids enter the blood, either directly from a sourdough bread soon after a meal, or by absorption from the colon several hours after a meal, they can be used directly as an energy source, and they tend to decrease the amount of insulin in the blood. This corresponds to a decrease in the glycemic effect, including reduced cholesterol levels. The presence of resistant starch and other soluble fiber will slow down the digestion of a bread. If the wholegrain flour is coarse, the slowed release of energy will be even greater than for a fine wholegrain flour, and a steadier energy flow should be felt all day.

Wholegrain rye has the full quota of nutrients to be expected from a wholegrain seed, including insoluble fiber and phenolics in the bran, starch and soluble-fiber pentosans in the endosperm, the B vitamins, enzymes, minerals, and phytic acid in the aleurone layer, and the valuable oils in the germ.

Sorghum

The Sudanese have relied on the sorghum grain for thousands of years and generally eat it in a fermented form, along with milk, or legume sauces called *mulahs,* which are made with cowpeas, lentils or peanuts, flavoring spices, and vegetables, such as tomato and onions, to make a more completely nutritious food. The low levels of lysine in the sorghum protein are compensated for by milk, legume sauce, or meat sauces. Sorghum is sprouted by the Sudanese to make it into malt, and since they are aware that poisonous hydrogen cyanide gas, dangerous to people, forms during the process, they know how to take preventive measures. The danger is unimportant for the sorghum malt itself because it is never consumed without being cooked, which eliminates the hydrogen cyanide gas. In addition, the young green leaves of sorghum are dangerous to cattle.

In dietary fiber, sorghum ranks among the highest of all the grains, and contains proportionately more than whole wheat. Insoluble fiber predominates, but 44 percent of its total fiber is soluble. Before sorghum is eaten, the husk is always removed, and sometimes the bran seed coat of the whole grain is also removed. It is important to know whether the sorghum you are eating is whole grain or not because the whole grain will contain large amounts of valuable fiber and all the associated vitamins and minerals, whereas the fractionated stripped sorghum will not.

Sorghum is rich in polyphenolic compounds that can bind to the starches and proteins released during digestion, and because these bound starches and proteins will not be digested until they reach the colon, they are effectively soluble fiber. This probably accounts for sorghum's exceptionally high-fiber value. In Africa, sorghum is traditionally made into a dough or a hot cereal that is fermented with a naturally occurring culture containing lactic bacteria and yeasts. When acids form during fermentation, the starch and protein bound to the polyphenolics is released and becomes digestible. Other advantages of fermentation include a better release of zinc and an increase in available niacin, riboflavin, and thiamine.

Sorghum has the reputation of not being fattening to animals or humans. The reason for this is its large amounts of polyphenolics that bind the starch and protein. By remaining undigested until reaching the colon, they release only half their caloric value, which was considered a disadvantage in the past, especially among those who used sorghum for animal food. On the other hand, the Sudanese people have thrived on sorghum prepared by traditional methods, and obesity and type-2 diabetes are basically unknown among them. The extremely high amounts of polyphenolics associated with fiber in sorghum lead to the probable conclusion that in all whole seed foods it is the polyphenolics that are partially responsible for reduced calories. By contrast, when refined wheat flour is made, most of the polyphenolics, along with the bran fiber, are removed from the wheat, which makes it more completely available for digestion and the resulting extra calories. Measuring the antioxidant value of a starchy food may turn out to be a means of evaluating its fattening power, and foods with a high content of antioxidant polyphenolics would be the least fattening.

Teff

One of the *lost* crops of Africa, teff (*Eragrostis tef*) is a wonderful grass that has survived as a staple food in Ethiopia throughout the millennia because it can grow under extreme conditions. Teff is now grown in Idaho and is widely available in North America, where it is especially popular with transplanted Ethiopians and those who cannot tolerate wheat-based foods. Due primarily to disastrous agricultural practices by non-Africans, African countries seem prone to famine, yet they have a rich heritage of crops that can produce good yields every year despite the fluctuations in rainfall. Information on many of these crops, including teff, has been collected in "The Lost Crops of Africa," a National Research Council (NRC) publication, which encourages their development and popularity. In impoverished regions of Africa, the rush to produce bumper crops of wheat along the lines of the Western world can be catastrophic when the wheat varieties planted must rely on expensive irrigation and fertilizer methods. There is also a great need to match agricultural methods with the prevailing climate in order to produce an adequate crop. Teff is still the preferred staple in Ethiopia because it survives the climate, and the Ethiopians know how to make a very popular injera bread from it. Teff has a really tiny seed, so the tasks of harvesting and separating the seed are very labor-intensive. This makes it expensive to produce, and there is always the temptation to look for cheaper grain foods, but so far, good sense has prevailed among the Ethiopians. Teff is a highly nutritious grain with an unusually high proportion of lysine in its protein, and is always eaten in the wholegrain form. Because the seed is so small, a very high proportion of fiber, especially insoluble fiber, is contributed by the bran seed coat (the ratio of insoluble fiber to soluble fiber is 4 to 1). Associated with the seed-coat fiber, aleurone layer, and germ are B vitamins, beta-carotenes, essential oils, and minerals. Fermentation during the preparation of the injera bread makes these nutrients highly available—iron-deficient anemia is practically unknown in areas where teff injera is the staple food.

Teff seeds can be white or chocolate-brown. As might be expected, the chocolate-colored teff has a richer flavor and even has a hint of chocolate flavor when made into injera bread. White teff is used to make a white injera bread and is generally reserved for special occasions, such as weddings.

Wheat

The large starchy endosperm in a grain of wheat can be completely separated from the nutrient-rich germ, the aleurone layer, and the bran by roller milling. This process was hailed as a major breakthrough in the 1880s before anyone knew about the B vitamins in the aleurone layer, the vitamin E in the germ, the many functions of fiber, or the antioxidant polyphenolics in the bran. The temptation to completely isolate the endosperm as refined white flour was, and is, very great. White flour is easy for bakers to work with, and they have learned to make some tantalizing white breads, cakes, pastries, and pies. All the careful research that has revealed the need to eat grains whole has had little impact, until now, when the effects of refined white flour are finally being graphically demonstrated by the huge number of people who are obese or have diabetes in the United States and Western Europe. Granted there are other causes for obesity, such as the general lack of adequate exercise, the acceptance of overly large serving portions in restaurants, and the almost universal consumption of sweetened soft drinks instead of water. Yet it is also obvious that, if every grain food is refined, it is providing many more calories than it would in the wholegrain form where the same portion would include fiber, which provides just half the calories of starch.

In many refined wheat flours, 76 percent of the original wheat grain that remains is almost pure endosperm. Gluten protein is associated with starch in the endosperm, in amounts that enable bakers to create white bread and cakes. Only a little fiber is present in the endosperm, and the cooking causes some of the starch to resist digestion until it reaches the microflora of the colon. This resistant starch produced in cooking is called dietary fiber, and is what allows wheat pastas and breads to contain more fiber than the flour from which they are made. It should be noted that attractive breads and pastas can be made with the bran and germ still in the flour, but the art of whole-wheat breadmaking has been neglected ever since the advent of roller milling. The art of wholegrain breadmaking, in general, is overdue for a strong revival now that we know so much more about the nutrients present in wholegrain flours.

Reviving Wholegrain Breadmaking. The revival of whole-wheat breadmaking, already making headway in major cities but lacking in most of the country, is dependent on the milling process for wheat. Fluffy, light-textured whole-wheat bread that is also healthy demands a whole-wheat flour that has plenty of fine particles, without pulverizing the bran and germ. The right degree of fineness can be felt by squeezing a handful of the flour—it forms a clump when there are enough really fine particles—and this is still best achieved by cool-stone milling. The skills needed to dress millstones and the mills themselves are rare, but they could be regained if minds and money were put to the task. The milling engineers who have so ingeniously produced refined flour could now apply their ingenuity to producing whole-wheat flour in the various degrees of fineness needed to make appealing whole-wheat breads.

Simply recombining the fractions of wheat obtained from roller milling does not produce a pleasing whole-wheat flour. The roller-milling process calls for the wheat to be initially moistened to aid in removing the bran. Moistening, or tempering, the wheat sets the enzymes (including fat-degrading enzymes) in motion for the wheat to sprout. As soon as these enzymes are active, the oils from the germ are broken down into their component acids and oxidized, resulting in a rancid flavor and the loss of nutritionally valuable oils during storage of the flour. The natural antioxidants present can offer great protection against rancidity, but only if the wheat grain is kept dry.

Whole-wheat flour made by cool-stone milling of wheat that has *never* been tempered by moistening can be kept for a long time with only slight changes in its vitamin and phytonutrient content (the actual storage time possible will depend on temperature and dryness). In a well-cooled grocery store, I have seen a shelf life of more than a year for some stone-milled whole-wheat flour. For bakers this should be a triumphant revelation.

Whole-wheat bread texture is improved if whole-wheat flour is stored for two weeks or longer at room temperature. In my own experience, the flavor of bread made from six-week-old whole-wheat flour is at least as good as if the flour was freshly ground. Old-fashioned porous cloth and paper bags may enhance the effects, compared with storage in plastic, even though most plastic is permeable to oxygen. A current theory to explain this phenomenon is that oxygen from the air is absorbed by the phenolic compounds. These oxidized phenolic compounds, which have been spread throughout the flour as a result of the milling, can form linkages with the gluten protein, and give a stronger gluten matrix to the bread. Still, for some bakers, freshly ground whole-wheat flour is unbeatable for its flavor.

Further consideration for the whole-wheat miller who would like to please whole-wheat bakers is the degree of starch damage. Starch damage sounds drastic, but is actually an expression to describe the rupturing of starch granules so they are able to absorb moisture nicely in a dough. These damaged starch granules are more readily degraded to simple sugars by the wheat enzymes, which are brought into action by moisture when bread dough is made.

Simple sugars are the energy food for yeasts and lactic bacteria that are used to ferment a bread dough successfully. No need to add sugar to the dough if there is enough damaged starch. Starch damage happens naturally when hard wheat is milled (but not at all for really soft wheat). The most common type is hard red wheat from the North American prairies. Bread from the softer wheats, which were popular before the 1880s and the advent of roller milling, have not been made in quantity since then. In fact, roller milling was invented to make use of the hard wheats that flourish in the climate and soil of the prairies.

Fortunately, there is no need for the miller to devise a way to produce enough damaged starch in flours. When soft wheats were more generally used in Western Europe for making breads, bakers were damaging the starch by first making a mash from a portion of the flour, a technique that fell from favor with the widespread use of refined flour and baker's yeast. Beermakers know about mashing grains with enzyme-active malt. The mash lasts one to three hours and the temperature is usually 60–70°C (140–158°F). Enzymes such as alpha-amylase and phytase are sped up, while beta-amylase and other enzymes are deactivated. Amylase can convert starch into simple sugars and sweet-tasting oligosaccharides that can be selectively used by the sourdough bacteria and yeasts. Phytase breaks down phytic acid into inositol and phosphate, and releases minerals. Making this mash by adding boiling water to flour, damages the starch too, so it is not necessary for the milling process to be the source of adequate damaged starch. The improvement in the bread by using a mash is particularly exciting for wholegrain breadmaking. Damaged starch, from the mash, can make a dough stiff enough to hold all the water required to fully hydrate the bran fiber and all the soluble fiber, and still stand up as a shaped bread. Fully hydrated bran will be so soft that it can no longer be accused of piercing, and ruining, the gluten structure of the bread.

The ultimate way to eat whole wheat is in the form of bread, but to achieve the pinnacle of nutritional advantage it should be leavened with a culture of compatible yeasts and lactic bacteria. Some of these yeasts and bacteria survive the baking process, and are carried all the way to the colon with the bran and soluble fiber. They can then favorably populate the colon, and keep it repopulated with lactic bacteria, as can the lactic bacteria from yogurt when regularly eaten. Soluble fiber and resistant starch also reach the colon, and aid in the multiplication of these favorable lactic bacteria which can break them down almost completely.

The short-chain acids that are made by fermenting soluble fiber in the colon have remarkably beneficial effects:

- The colon is well acidified by the short-chain fatty acids, which keep unfavorable microorganisms to a minimum, and reduce vulnerability to colon cancer;

- The absorption of the short-chain fatty acids leads to a reduction in cholesterol;

- Colonic fermentation leads to the release of antioxidant phenolic compounds from the fiber and their absorption, which partly explains the protection against coronary heart disease among people who eat whole-wheat bread (in general, protection against heart disease is greater from whole grains than from fruits and vegetables).

Natural Sourdough. This dough contains a mixture of compatible yeasts and lactic bacteria, and even though there is a mystique surrounding the leavening ingredients, the fact is, bakeries make consistently good bread using natural sourdough—these bakeries bask in the delicious aroma produced by their sourdough breads with their characteristic taste. The most robust, natural sourdough leavenings are maintained with a wholegrain flour, usually wheat or rye, and a small amount of added malted wheat or barley to complete the needs of the microorganisms. The malt should be made from sprouted grain, which has been oven-dried at a low enough temperature to preserve the enzymes. When the sourdough is made with a mash of wholegrain flour and enzyme-active malt, it is essentially the same as the old-fashioned Celtic *barm,* or sweet sourdough. Barm breadmaking is reputed to be the ancient Egyptian way of making bread, according to William Jago in 1911. It's time to revive the word *barm* and the *barm* process, alongside the revival of wholegrain breadmaking. Baker's yeast was invented in the 1800s, specifically for use with refined white flours. It is incompatible with lactic bacteria because they both use the same nutrients. For this reason, any sourdough made with baker's yeast will have fewer lactic bacteria than are found in natural sourdough.

Other Wheat-Based Foods. Although the main destination for wheat grains is flour for baked goods, wheat is also eaten as a breakfast cereal, a whole-kernel grain in soups and tabbouleh salad, and of course, pasta. The wheat flour for pasta is usually refined endosperm flour, only a few producers currently make 100-percent whole-wheat pasta. For breakfast cereals, wheat is often kept whole, but there are several wheat cereals where the bran only is eaten, or the endosperm alone is eaten as a hot cereal.

Unlike bread, the wheat in cold cereals is much more often wholegrain. People who eat these cereals for breakfast in moderate portions are more likely to have a healthy weight than those who skip breakfast altogether, or those who eat a meat-and-egg type of breakfast, as proven by a large group studied between 1988 and 1994 and reported in the Third National Health and Nutrition Survey in 2003. All of this demonstrates that we need to know how much wholegrain wheat is in our food so we can recognize its true nutritional contribution to our well-being.

By far the greatest proportion of fiber in wheat is found in the bran seed coat—this bran fiber is mostly insoluble, with smaller amounts of soluble fiber. Wheat bran is the best source of insoluble fiber and is an essential laxative. Within the bran fiber matrix are polyphenolic compounds that give it color and flavor and act as powerful antioxidants and UV-light absorbers. Red wheat bran has more antioxidant power than white wheat bran, but both can help protect people from arteriosclerosis and other degenerative diseases. The polyphenolics released in the colon as a result of bacterial enzymes offer anti-cancer protection in the colon. In France, people eat sufficient amounts of bran-fiber cereal to see that it has a protective effect against breast cancer. In the United States, such correlations have not been seen because it is so difficult to know how much bran and whole grains there are in commercial American baked goods and cereals.

Also closely associated with the bran fiber is the aleurone layer, the B vitamins (B_6, biotin, folate, niacin, pantothenate, riboflavin, and thiamine) and the minerals that it contains in valuable amounts. Sufficient amounts of certain B vitamins are essential for a well-regulated release of energy from starch—so much so that the major B vitamins (niacin, riboflavin, and thiamine) are deliberately added back to refined white endosperm flour, which lacks the aleurone layer.

Whole Wheat vs. Refined Wheat Flours. In the late 1920s, refined flour was the main winter provision for a group of fishermen in Newfoundland who were cut off from supplies of fresh foods, and the deficiency disease beriberi was common among them. As mentioned earlier, this disease is usually associated with a lack of thiamine from a polished rice diet, but refined wheat also lacks thiamine and can lead to this disease. There were many other examples of beriberi outbreaks in North America resulting from a restricted diet of refined wheat flour, especially among the poor in the South. Similarly in 1916, while under siege by the Turks, British soldiers eating white bread succumbed to beriberi, while the East Indians with them did not because they were eating whole-wheat chapattis.

According to legend, in 1812 the village of Borodino just outside Moscow managed to hold out against the French under Napoleon during their march on Moscow because the Russian soldiers were supplied with the specially baked black whole rye and wheat breads typical of the town. This bread has been famous ever since as borodinski bread. These and similar stories, including those told by Sylvester Graham in his *Treatise on Bread and Bread Making,* predate our knowledge of vitamins, but confirm that the benefits of wholegrain breads have always been appreciated by observant thinkers.

In the middle-class South London suburbs of the 1950s, the results of thiamine deficiency were brought home to me by my mother. She had just learned, while out shopping, that a distinctly overweight neighbor of ours had been diagnosed with beriberi. Thinking beriberi was a historical disease typical of poor eaters of white rice, I found this news shocking, as well as educational. I later learned that thiamine can be drastically reduced in scones and cakes when baking soda is used as a leavening agent, because the alkaline nature of the soda breaks down the thiamine. By then, both in Britain and the United States, white flour was at least enriched with thiamine, riboflavin, niacin, and iron, so she must have been eating scones and cakes rather than yeasted bread, and little of anything else. Yeast-leavened breads do not damage the thiamine as seriously, and sourdough-leavened breads are sufficiently acidic that the thiamine is stabilized against the heat of cooking.

In wheat, phytic acid is present in the bran and aleurone layers, and is a source of phosphate for the developing plant, but it diminishes in sprouting wheat seeds, as well as when whole-wheat flours are fermented in a dough. Phytic acid is a beneficial nutrient that has been associated with protection against colon cancer, and recently a reduced risk for kidney stones. Any adverse effects of phytic acid (it can cause mineral deficiencies) disappear when the wheat seed is soaked, sprouted, or fermented, especially with a sourdough containing lactic bacteria and a compatible yeast.

The fiber in wheat germ is significant and contains a higher proportion of soluble fiber than bran, as might be imagined for a plant embryo. Essential fatty acids, vitamin-E tocopherols, and a rich supply of folic acid are all concentrated in the oils of wheat germ, and all are necessary nutrients for healthy cell multiplication in plants, as well as in people. Along with the fiber, phytic acid and other valuable phytonutrients, such as polyphenolics, are contained in wheat germ. Additionally, the germ is naturally very rich in folic acid, a nutrient now recognized as protective against high homocysteine levels in the blood—low homocysteine levels in the blood are associated with a low risk for Alzheimer's disease and heart disease. Wheat germ is also very rich in betaine, another compound capable of lowering homocysteine levels. Both betaine and folate, as well as the antioxidant polyphenolics in the bran, are contributing to wholegrain wheat's reputation of being more protective against heart disease than even fruits and vegetables.

Wheat comes in many varieties. The wheat used for breadmaking should have more than 12-percent protein, and preferably more than 14 percent, as should the durum wheat for pasta. Some of the more exotic wheats include einkorn, farro, Kamut, and spelt, which are frequently available in wholegrain form. All provide insoluble bran fiber and the associated soluble fiber just below the bran, both of which are valuable for a healthy colon and healthy elimination habits. Provided they are eaten as a wholegrain staple, the particular value of wheat and rye is the relatively large amounts of nutrients that can be eaten at every meal. When they are, the result is a constant replenishment of grain fiber, vitamins, minerals, and other phytonutrients that are protective against arterial disease, cancer, and diabetes, and generally contribute to our well-being.

With the current awareness of wholegrain flour's benefits, it is almost unthinkable that refined white flour is still the mainstay of the American diet. In the 1990s, when all-natural artisanal breads were promoted, the thrust was towards organic flour without bleach. Certainly, eliminating the bleach, with its possible carcinogenic byproducts, was an admirable approach. But the unbleached flour was still refined, and in their zeal to produce bread from organic flour without additives, many of the artisans failed to enrich it with vitamins. These artisans are lucky to have catered to the affluent who could afford a varied diet, or there might have been renewed outbreaks of beriberi and pellagra among any poor people who had to subsist on such bread. Fortunately, there are now a number of artisanal bakers who devote their energies to making 100-percent organic *wholegrain* breads. More of *these* bakers are needed, and it is important to support and encourage them instead of the bakers who, although using organic flour for their good-looking boutique products, are still providing unhealthful, refined-flour breads.

18

What's with Fiber in Beans and Legumes?

Beans—One Key to a Successful Plant-Based Diet

Western diets would be much more nutritious and exciting if beans and legumes were used more, but at least there are Boston baked beans, great Northern bean soups, and multi-bean salads. Eastern Mediterranean cooks make delicious sesame and chickpea dishes, Mexicans have bean burritos, and East Indians make excellent lentil curries. In Scandinavia, split pea soups are eaten regularly, the Chinese make a sweetened bean-paste filling for buns, and the Japanese make miso, a fermented bean paste made from soybeans and eaten as a soup. The soybean has been commandeered from Asia, but aside from being grown for animal feed, it is mostly extracted for its oil, or its protein is made into tofu.

Nuts and seeds are the plant world's suppliers of oils and proteins, grains provide mostly starch with some protein, and legumes (beans, lentils, peanuts, and peas) provide protein, some starch, and sometimes oil. The amino-acid profiles of the proteins in each group are often complementary so that, when eaten together, the combined protein profile is similar to a complete protein found only in animal foods. Eating nuts and legumes, as well as grains, all in the whole form, provides a sound basis for a plant-based diet—complementary proteins, digestible carbohydrates, fiber, oils, and phytonutrients.

It is really possible to have an exciting diet based on plant foods, but there is one essential proviso, namely that the grains, nuts, seeds, and legumes are eaten in the whole form. Only then is it possible to derive enough nourishment without resorting to large amounts of meat for fat, protein, and a supply of the B vitamins. Many people successfully eat a whole plant-based diet with the addition of eggs, cheese, and milk, and in some cases a little flesh protein, usually in the form of chicken or fish. Too large an amount of these animal products, however, will make too little space on the plate for the plant foods, together with their fiber, which offer so much when eaten in the whole form.

Beans, peas, lentils, and peanuts all belong to the legume plant family. The legume's classification is useful because all the legumes have a high protein content that is complementary to the protein from grains. The combination of grains and beans results in a more nutritious complete protein than could be supplied by either beans or grains alone.

Beans are the single most nutritious, yet neglected, food in today's sophisticated lifestyle. People make all sorts of excuses for omitting beans from their diet, and they are almost never offered in European-style restaurants. Sadly, beans are still considered the food of the poor, or unsophisticated. Bean salads do appear in American restaurants, usually as a buffet item, and of course beans are definitely on the menu of Mexican restaurants. In North American restaurants, 100-percent wholegrain breads and bean dishes are rarely served. Their absence often makes restaurant visits very disappointing to us, since we like to eat a legume dish daily for dinner, and accompany a salad with wholegrain bread, both of which are worthy of the chef's imagination, in our opinion.

Learning to Eat Precious Beans

Beyond the image of poverty and lack of sophistication, perhaps the most embarrassing reason for not eating beans is that they can cause flatulence (gas). Amazing as it may seem, the most successful cure for flatulence is to eat beans daily and always as part of a meal rather than alone as a snack. Beans are rich in soluble fiber, which of course remains undigested until it reaches the bacteria in the colon and is fermented. The bacteria become accustomed to the soluble bean fiber, and those bacteria capable of using the bean fiber without making a gas increasingly predominate; the process takes about two weeks, but once that embarrassment is overcome, the benefits are wonderful—a truly delicious food is added to your diet, and there is a subsequent reduction in your LDL cholesterol from the soluble fiber, to mention only two of the many benefits.

Another bonus that comes with beans is a generous proportion of *insoluble* fiber that simply serves to hold moisture and carry your food all the way through your system. A daily serving of beans, and several servings of 100-percent wholegrain foods provides enough insoluble fiber to guarantee the requisite one-to-two day transit time for complete freedom from constipation. It is very difficult to supply enough daily fiber to achieve this without resorting to a supplement unless beans and whole grains are included in your diet.

The benefits of eating beans also include a rich supply of folate and potassium. It's not at all surprising that it became necessary to add folate to refined white flour because the two major sources of folate are wheat germ and beans. Wheat germ is discarded from refined white flour and beans are too often ignored. The potassium in legumes and other plant foods acts as a natural regulator of blood pressure. People who eat a whole plant-based diet, including beans daily, and who also avoid oversalting food, are less likely to need medication to control their blood pressure.

Botanically, legume seeds have two food-storage organs called cotyledons, which are the bean or pea halves that break apart when the skin is removed. (*See* Figures 18.1 and 18.2.) Cotyledons have different properties and structure than the endosperm storage organ of the grass family seeds, such as barley, oats, rye, and wheat. Cotyledons are leaf-like in structure and even grow out of the legume seed on the stem, to be above ground. In the cotyledons, the cell-wall materials (fiber) are distributed throughout with the protein, oils, starch, sugars, and other phytonutrients that are inside each of the minute cells. This contrasts with wheat where the endosperm storage organ has very little cell structure, and therefore very little fiber, and is mainly built from starch granules. Even if the skin is removed from beans, there is still a high proportion of the total fiber and accompanying nutrients remaining in the cotyledons.

Old World Beans and Peas

History classifies legumes as either Old or New World. Known since ancient times, the Old World beans and peas include the peas (*Pisum*) from Europe,

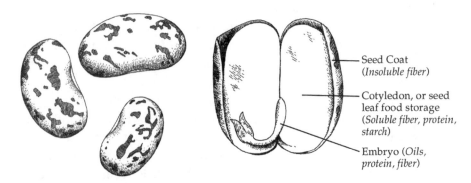

Figure 18.1. Whole Beans   **Figure 18.2.** Open Bean

Seed Coat (*Insoluble fiber*)

Cotyledon, or seed leaf food storage (*Soluble fiber, protein, starch*)

Embryo (*Oils, protein, fiber*)

cowpeas *(Vigna)* from Africa, lentils *(Lens),* mung, black gram, and adzuki *(Phaseolus aureus, P. mungo,* and *P. angularis* respectively) beans from Asia, chickpeas *(Cicer),* lupine *(Lupinus),* and fava *(Vicia)* beans from the Mediterranean region and beyond, and soybeans *(Glycine maximus)* from China and Japan.

Peas

In Britain and the Scandinavian countries, peas are a regular, welcome vegetable. The favorite ways to eat them are as whole-pod peas, vegetable peas, dried whole peas, and split peas. Before the seeds mature, whole-pod peas are eaten early in the season, then the green peas are favored, and finally the fully dried peas can be stored for pea soups.

The whole pod supplies an expected amount of fiber, mostly insoluble, but with enough soluble fiber to benefit your cholesterol profile. Once the peas have matured and are eaten separately from the pod, the pea skin contributes a high proportion of fiber. Dried whole peas retain the skin, but dried split peas do not, so the fiber in those is somewhat reduced. Even so, split peas can contribute to the day's fiber because the main structure of the pea in the cotyledons contains a considerable amount of it, along with protein and starch. The embryo remains attached to the split peas and contains minerals, including potassium, and the B vitamins, especially folic acid.

Brown rice and peas is a frequent combination that enhances the protein value of both the rice and the peas. Brown rice is the rice of choice, naturally, since it is nutritionally superior to white rice and has a much more interesting flavor.

Cowpeas

Black-eyed peas are the most familiar example of cowpeas. African in origin, they were probably brought to America by the Spaniards and the slave traders, and were enjoyed by Thomas Jefferson and Mark Twain alike. In Southern soul food, black-eyed peas, along with pork, are an important ingredient. Carolina Hoppin' John is a combination of cowpeas, rice, and a ham bone, which illustrates the instinctive complementary mixing of legume and grain. Having personally learned that the full flavor of cooked beans does not require the fat or bone of meat, it is never added in our house. Olive oil is, however, added after the peas have been cooked. Black-eyed peas are prepared whole, complete with their thin fiber skin, and as with all legumes, black-eyed peas supply protein, starch, some oils, the requisite fiber, minerals, and B vitamins to maintain the body, and the soul.

Lentils

With their beautiful green or orange-red color, lentils are eyecatchers and a reminder that protective phytonutrients are present. The color disappears when they are cooked, but the compounds in the phytonutrients are only diluted by the water that is absorbed. Orange-red lentils are frequently the basis of Ethiopian stews (w'et) that are eaten with teff injera bread. Green lentils beg for the spices of Indian cooking—chili pepper, coriander, cumin, fenugreek, garlic, ginger, mustard, onions, and turmeric—used selectively, and generally in moderation, but occasionally very hotly. All are rich in antioxidants that add to the already healthy value of the lentils.

Lentils are often cooked with rice, thereby enhancing the value of the protein. In American cooking, lentils are usually combined with carrots, celery, garlic, onion, tomato, and vinegar. Lentil fiber, both soluble and insoluble, is plentiful in the green lentils especially, and these are eaten with the seed coat on. There is a little less fiber with orange-red lentils because they are normally eaten without the seed coat. Of all the legumes, lentils supply the greatest concentration of folate.

Mung, Black Gram, and Adzuki Beans

The mung bean (*Phaseolus aureus*) is a small green-colored bean, primarily grown to produce sprouts. In China, mung sprouts are often sautéed with other vegetables, such as onions, and are an ingredient in many dishes, including Chinese cellophane noodles. Sprouting increases the B-vitamin content, and the soluble fiber.

The mung bean is called *P. aureus,* and the black gram *P. mungo.* The latter is a small black bean famous in India for its use as an ingredient in idli and dosa rice cakes.

In China and Japan, the adzuki bean (*P. angularis*) is almost as commercially important as the soybean. Although used for savory bean dishes of all kinds, adzuki beans are the beans of choice for desserts where they are made into a paste for filling pastries and adding to ice cream.

All the nutritional advantages of beans—a high ratio of potassium to sodium, magnesium, and the B vitamins (folic acid in particular) can be found in the mung, the black gram, and the adzuki beans.

Chickpeas/Garbanzo Beans

Because chickpeas are our favorite legume, we eat them on Sundays, holidays, and often on birthdays and anniversaries too. Some varieties are small and have a dark skin, but most now are quite large and thin-skinned and will cook to a soft consistency very well. These chickpeas are so delicately and sweetly flavored that they can be prepared and enjoyed with a just a little salt and pepper. In keeping with their 7,000 year history, beginning in Egypt, however, there are some classic chickpea dishes, such as Middle-Eastern hummus, that are also current favorites. Hummus is a combination of tahini paste (ground sesame seeds), cooked chickpeas, garlic, and lemon that is usually served with trimmed vegetables for dipping, and pita bread. Japanese miso can be made by fermenting chickpeas instead of soybeans and barley, and the result is a remarkable milder, sweeter, instant-soup base.

Chickpea flour is used in several countries. In Greece it is used as a rusk ingredient. In Persia they make a shortbread with it. The Italians make a thin pancake, and in India, they make a fritter. Roasted chickpeas are fabulous in trail mix, or as a snack, with raisins and almonds. Before we knew of such a delicacy, a thoughtful friend once gave us some lightly roasted chickpeas as a gift, which surprised us almost as much as their light crunchy texture and sweet flavor did. To prepare roasted chickpeas by the Indian method, boil chickpeas in water until tender but still holding their shape, and then drain and lightly roast them. Add salt and flavorings later.

The Italians remove the skins of chickpeas after they have been cooked. The chickpeas are placed between two cloths and a rolling pin is rolled over them. Perhaps this was the method applied to the dark-skinned variety, because the chickpeas with a fairly thin and translucent skin that are available today are easily eaten, with no rolling pin required.

Whole cooked chickpeas are as nutritionally reliable as other beans. They supply plenty of fiber, soluble and insoluble, and their main nutrients, starch, protein, and a little oil, are in good balance. The B vitamins, particularly folic acid, are well supplied, as are minerals, including potassium and the antioxidant polyphenolics.

Lupine Beans

Lupine beans are not much eaten in North America, although they are often available in Italian specialty stores. It had always been our impression that lupine seeds were poisonous, so the discovery of Italian lupine beans came as a surprise. Apparently non-poisonous varieties were developed in the 1920s, and prior to that time special cooking techniques were used to remove the bitter-tasting alkaloids. The raw beans are given a twelve-hour soaking, followed by a rinsing before cooking, and after cooking they are stored and rinsed in salted water for six or seven days, until no bitterness remains. In Roman times, vast quantities of lupine beans were eaten, especially by the poor, but New World beans have become so popular, they are rarely eaten now.

Fava Beans

Fava beans now seem to be the farmers' favorite winter legume cover crop here in California, where they get ploughed under to nourish the soil rather than people. A few fava beans survive, however, to make it to the lunch table as a salad, sautéed with garlic, and dressed with lemon and olive oil, and some even are served as dinner beans. The sixth-century B.C. philosopher, Pythagoras, shunned fava beans, and since his time it's been discovered that some people cannot tolerate them. In susceptible people, fava beans induce anemia and jaundice, an effect known as favism. Fava beans are quite large, and when mature it is possible to remove the thick, highly flavored skins before cooking them. The bean skin is particularly rich in polyphenolic compounds, which explains the strong flavor and is a good reason to eat the whole bean—the bean center is much more delicately textured and flavored. With the whole bean, there is a good supply of folic acid and other B vitamins. A type of fava bean in Egypt is used to make *Ful medames*, their national dish. In Britain, the broad bean is another type of fava bean that I do not recall having such a strong flavor as the ones here in California, probably because they were harvested and dried before they were fully matured.

Soybeans

The outstanding characteristics of soybeans are their high oil content, high protein (more than 35 percent), and relatively small amount of starch or sugar. The oil is particularly rich in lecithin and vitamin-E tocopherols. Soybeans have also made the news with their anti-cancer isoflavones, which are described more generally as polyphenolics.

Soy protein is built from a well-balanced mixture of amino acids, which makes it very similar, nutritionally, to animal protein. Both soluble and insoluble fiber is there, of course, in the cotyledons and skin of the soybean. In regions of Southeast Asia, China, and Japan, where relatively little meat is eaten, the soybean is a very important staple food. Cooking soybeans by first soaking, then boiling them until tender, takes a long time and is necessary to deactivate the digestive inhibitors present in raw soybeans, so this is not the most popular preparation method. The more prevalent process for soybeans begins by removing the bean skin and then grinding the soybean to a flour. In water, the soy flour cooks easily in thirty minutes. An even better method is to grind soaked soybeans into boiling water and finish the cooking after that, which dissipates the strong soybean flavor. Soy milk is made from these ground, cooked soybeans by straining off the milky liquid. The remaining residue, known as okara, is also eaten. Tofu is made from soy milk by adding a calcium-sulfate solution which precipitates the tofu curds of protein and fat.

Soybeans eaten in the form of soy milk and tofu are not whole—most of the fiber is left in the okara residue. In Asia it is likely that soy milk, tofu, and okara are all eaten, so the separations result in little loss of the original whole soybean nutrients. There must be some loss of nutrients in the whey, which is produced when tofu curds are separated and pressed into a tofu block. Nevertheless, it appears that cancers and heart disease are much reduced in Southeast Asia, and this is attributed to the large amounts of soy products and associated phytochemicals in the diet. Although the active phytochemicals (saponins and polyphenolics) are concentrated in the embryo of the soybean, processing seems to release them, and allows them to be trapped by the protein in the production of soy milk and tofu. Most beans possess a generous supply of these phytochemicals, but soy has been the most highly studied. The okara probably has the highest concentration of these phytochemicals because the fiber is concentrated here. Soybean skins have, so far, not been found to contain any particularly healthful phytonutrients, so it does not seem to matter that they are discarded.

Sprouting soybeans is a way to enhance the vitamin and fiber content and also deactivate some of the digestive inhibitors. Soybean sprouts are cooked before eating, so the deactivation of the digestive inhibitors is completed.

Tempeh, a Fermented Soybean Product

One of the most nutritious ways to eat whole soybeans is in the form of fermented tempeh. Soybeans are first boiled, then the skins are removed and they are split into halves. When the soybeans are drained and cool, they are inoculated with the mold *Rhizopus oligosporus* and allowed to ferment at approximately 90°F. Within twenty-four hours, this mold grows throughout the soybeans and binds them together into a thin solid cake. The result is a deliciously savory, highly nutritious food that is especially good when eaten fresh. Tempeh should *always* be cooked, since the soybeans used in the preparation are not cooked sufficiently at the beginning to inactivate the digestive inhibitors present in all raw beans, including soybeans. The fermentation produces vitamin B_{12}, a rare vitamin for a plant food, and especially useful for vegans who do not eat any animal products. (There is, however, a scientific controversy as to whether this B_{12} is in a usable form.) The methionine amino-acid content of the protein is also increased by the fermentation, which makes the soy protein even more completely assimilated. As in other legumes, soybeans are also high in the amino acid lysine, and this makes it an ideal complement to the wheat in breads. Tempeh is a soybean food that includes all the nutrients of the whole bean. All the fiber is present, along with the protein, oil, starch, vitamins, minerals, and phytonutrients, plus a full measure of isoflavones.

Miso for Sauces and Soups

Miso is another fermented soybean product utilizing whole soybeans that are thoroughly soaked and cooked without their skins, and are sometimes ground to grits beforehand. Rice and barley are often incorporated in making miso and they too are fermented, but separately, before being added to the soybeans for the final ferment. Miso is, above all, a soup base, and there are variations in style from mild to salty and tangy. (Other beans are also made into miso, the most notable being chickpea miso, which is made up without the addition of any other grain or bean. It makes a wonderful lunch soup that can be served with dulse seaweed to emulate the Japanese style of serving miso with seaweed.) The nutrients in miso soybeans are modified by the fermentation. The protein content is enhanced and the starch is decreased, and among the products of the fermentation are enzymes that digest proteins and starches, riboflavin (vitamin B_2), a strong antioxidant protector of vitamin A, and vitamin B_{12}.

Various soy sauces are also produced by fermenting a mixture of soybeans and roasted whole wheat. These sauces lack the soybean fiber, but during the fermentation process, many of the antioxidant polyphenolics are released from both the wheat and the soybeans. They are also very strongly flavored and colored, and contribute to the soy-sauce flavor. All the fermentations of soybeans lead to modified amino acids from the proteins, including glutamic acid, which naturally gives deliciousness, or *umami*, to well-made soy sauces.

New World Beans

New World beans, indigenous to the American continent, were brought to Spain, and from there to the rest of the world, following Columbus' voyage in 1492. New World beans are referred to as haricots in France, hence the French name *haricots vert* for cut green beans. At least four categories of New World beans or haricots are recognized. The most popular New World beans (*Phaseolus vulgaris*) have a wide range of appearances, and include black, cannellini, cranberry, flageolet, great Northern, kidney, navy, and pinto beans. The most common group of New World bean is the lima bean *(Phaseolus lunatus)* from Peru. Runner (string) beans in a large pod from vividly red flowers are in the *Phaseolus coccineus* group. Tepary beans *(Phaseolus acutifolius)* are still quite rare. Some tepary beans look like kidney beans, but are distinctive because the plants are drought-tolerant and can be grown in desert conditions.

Popular New World Beans (Phaseolus vulgaris)

The most popular beans that originated on the American continent vary greatly in color and to a lesser extent in flavor. The darkest colored black beans and the red kidney beans have the most powerful flavor. The variegated pinto and cranberry beans are milder, but not so delicate in flavor as the white, navy, or great Northern beans. Black beans are also known as black turtle beans and are important in Mexican cooking. Traditionally, white navy beans are used to make Boston baked beans. Some have been adopted by European countries as a very appetizing alternative to the fava bean, the best example being the white cannellini bean adopted by the Italians.

All these New World beans can be soaked and cooked by boiling in water. Flavoring is added only after the beans are fully cooked. Early addition of salt, or acids, such as vinegar or lemon juice, seems to prevent the beans from cooking to complete softness. They are eaten as the whole cooked bean, including the skin, which is usually tender and unobtrusive in flavor. Because they are generally quite mild in flavor, they lend themselves to a range of bean dishes. Vegetarians relish them daily. Perhaps their rare presence at the meat eater's table is because they can be eaten *instead* of meat at dinner. Beans are exceptionally satisfying as a vegetable. Throughout America, beans are used to spread the available meat when it is in meager supply, in the dish chili for example. To be equivalent to meat, in terms of the amino acids in bean protein, a wholegrain food should be eaten with the beans, preferably at the same meal. Nuts and seeds, such as sesame, also complement beans and grains. Together they contribute all the essential amino acids in satisfactory amounts. In her book *Diet for a Small Planet,* Frances Moore Lappé describes this complementation in detail. She educated her generation, and beyond, on the possibilities of a vegetarian diet, and the ways in which it could benefit people and the planet. The benefit arises when whole plants—beans, grains, nuts, and small seeds—are eaten. Farming is better balanced and therefore more readily sustained without the excesses of mass meat production. The temptation toward massive production is fueled by shortcuts that are rarely in tune with the natural world.

By eating a portion of whole beans daily, nicely cooked and flavored of course, a very significant amount of fiber is ingested. The amount of fiber, mostly insoluble, is 12–17 grams, which is quite a generous contribution to the desired 35–50 grams of fiber daily. The soluble fiber contributes to the maintenance of low levels of LDL cholesterol. Polyphenols and phytates are associated with the fiber and contribute anti-cancer activity. Soybeans have been given the most research attention, but it is reasonable to suppose that all the New World beans possess several potent antioxidant phytonutrients. They certainly supply plenty of folic acid and potassium, as well as the other B vitamins and minerals.

Lima Beans *(Phaseolus lunatus)*

Lima beans originated in Peru, with its capital in Lima, which accounts for their name. In Britain, they are popular as butter beans, and are the size of fava beans, but much nicer to eat. According to a Peruvian friend, there are some large and delicious varieties she has seen for sale only in Peru, which suggest there are still plenty of bean varieties to seek out and enjoy. There is fiber in Lima beans, too, along with anti-cancer phenolic antioxidants, folic acid, B vitamins, and potassium to offset sodium intake and stabilize blood pressure, plus all those other known and unknown nutrients that give beans the power to help maintain good health.

A few varieties of Lima beans coming from the Caribbean contain toxic substances (cyanogenic glycosides). Fortunately, however, the soaking and cooking process drives these volatile toxic substances out of the beans, making them safe to eat.

Peanuts *(Arachis hypogaea)*

It's hard to imagine that the peanut, which originated in tropical South America, is no relation to the sophisticated almond or walnut. It is, in fact, a legume seed that behaves just like all the other beans and peas: when the skin is removed, the two cotyledons separate, revealing the small embryo root and shoot between them. Split peas and split peanuts are, after all, a product of their natural structure rather than a machine. The thin brown coat on the peanut is edible, and supplies some insoluble fiber and accompanying polyphenolics. Thiamin is concentrated in or just beneath the skin, and is the vitamin most easily lost from peanuts as a result of skin removal or roasting. As with all the legumes, there is also a generous supply of both soluble and insoluble fiber in the cotyledons (the food-storage units of the seed), and there is fiber in the embryo root and shoot. In general, legumes contain only a small amount of oil, but peanuts (especially) and soybeans are notable exceptions that contain a large proportion of oil. The oil content of roasted peanuts is 50 percent. The oil is distributed in the cotyledons in association with the fiber (7 percent), a generous amount of protein (20 percent), and an unusually small proportion of digestible carbohydrates, such as starches and sugars (both 6 percent). Peanuts in the form of roasted peanut butter, without any additives or modification, are a good source of B vitamins, especially folate and niacin, minerals, such as potassium and magnesium, and vitamin E associated with the high oil content. The oil is 50-percent monounsaturated, with a fairly high proportion (35 percent) being polyunsaturated, and the remaining 15 percent saturated. The protein value is enhanced when peanut butter is eaten with wholegrain bread. So, peanut butter that is well-produced, without pesticides, modifications, or additives, is indeed good food associated with its own inherent fiber. It is healthiest when made from freshly roasted peanuts that are freshly ground into peanut butter.

George Washington Carver was not the first to discover the food value and appetizing flavor of roasted peanuts, but he was instrumental in the invention and popularization of peanut butter in North America, starting about 1890.

An Ancient Food of the American Continent

As early as 2000 B.C., at least, peanuts were being grown in Peru and it is believed that they originated in the Amazon basin of Brazil and Paraguay. The Portuguese explorers of South America introduced them into East Africa, and peanuts arrived in North America with the slave trade. The Spanish explorers introduced them into the Philippines and Europe, and following that, they were introduced into most regions of the world where climates were suited to their cultivation. Some countries, such as Indonesia and Mali in East Africa, have developed an especially delicious cuisine with their peanut sauces.

Here in North America, the states with the most appropriate climate for peanuts are Alabama, Georgia, North Carolina, and Texas, so I was amazed when, one January, Gene brought home some freshly dug peanuts from our local farmers' market just south of San Francisco. The California winter is certainly mild, and the right rain pattern to keep the ground nicely moist for the previous six weeks had just occurred. The fresh peanuts looked and felt more like tiny potatoes, but with a waist. Aware of the aflatoxins from molds that can grow on peanuts if they are stored moist, we immediately dried them in our food dryer, and they looked exactly like peanuts in pods, with the familiar basket-weave pattern on the outside, and the two thin-skinned peanuts inside. Light roasting is the ultimate drying method for peanuts after they have been shelled, and is a necessary step for a reasonably prolonged storage of peanuts. Roasting renders the skin so fine and thin that it is usually removed, leaving the cream-colored halves of the peanuts devoid of brown skin. When oil is extracted from these peanuts, the residual paste contains most of the original nutrients, including the fiber. As it is, this paste can be made into cookies, but it is more usually sold as an additive for processed baked goods, and as an animal feed.

The widespread use of peanut butter and peanut oil has revealed that some people can have severely allergic reactions to peanuts. However, for many others, peanuts, especially in the form of peanut butter, are a welcome and readily available food.

Runner (String) Beans (*Phaseolus coccineus*)

The most striking feature of runner-bean plants, after the sheer height they climb, is the striking red flower. This could easily have been the bean made famous by the nursery tale of *Jack and the Beanstalk.* The beans are large and dramatically speckled in red and black, with a little white, and are often eaten in their whole tender green pods, as string beans before they have filled out and ripened. But, it is the mature runner-bean seed that has the full nutritional value to be expected from beans. The fiber, soluble and insoluble, is of great value, along with the protein and phytonutrients typical of the legume seed.

19

What's with Fiber in Nuts?

Nuts appear on dining tables as dessert treats: almond filling for pastries; almond marzipan on cakes and in Scandinavian cookies; chestnuts, hazelnuts, and walnuts in cake; pistachio nuts in ice cream; and, in Hawaii, macadamia nuts in a sweet pancake sauce. But it's time to treat nuts with greater respect as basic food. Nuts are seeds rich in the B and E vitamins, oils, and protein, and can be a valuable addition to trail mix with dried fruits. Nut milk, particularly almond milk, is an ancient food that originated in Persia and was popular all over Europe, especially in the Middle Ages.

Almonds

Up until the 1989 Loma Prieta earthquake here in the San Francisco Bay area, I used to blanch almonds for almond cookies. I remember the year exactly because Gene was talking to the participants in one of his clinical studies in a nearby hotel, and was giving out grocery bags of selected foods to be eaten with almonds exactly when the earthquake struck, and I was at home. While the earthquake waves rolled under the house, I took shelter under the dining table, quaking as the doorbell chimes clanged, and the bookcases crashed one by one like dominoes in the back room. As you can imagine, I felt the need to check on my husband's safety and ventured out to the nearby hotel where the meeting was being held, while the light poles in the parking lot were still swaying and the ground was still gently rolling. When I arrived at the hotel, my intrepid husband, Gene, behaved as though nothing at all extraordinary had happened. The study subjects had ducked under the slender tables, but Gene was continuously dispensing instructions on what to eat with the almonds during the study all through the most vigorous shaking I've ever encountered. Even so, it turned out to be a landmark study, which showed that whole almonds eaten as part of a whole plant-based diet could lower cholesterol. The initial prediction had been that the good fats in almonds would cause a reduction in cholesterol levels, but the results were so striking they suggested that other factors were involved. The almond skins with their rich supply of polyphenolics had helped to produce a dramatic reduction in cholesterol levels in just two weeks. Even more exciting, it was only the bad LDL cholesterol that was reduced, leaving the good HDL unchanged. Another factor that contributed to the effect was the protein in almonds, which is high in the amino acid arginine.

Whole almonds have had the hard woody shell removed (*see* Figures 19.2 and 19.2). The outermost skin of the whole almond is brown, mostly insoluble fiber, but it is associated with polyphenolic compounds that easily leach out into water. The polyphenolics in almonds will bind with sufficient starch and protein to carry them all the way to the colon before being released by the lactic bacteria. The general availability of the nutrients in the almonds will, of course, depend on whether they have been left whole or have been chopped or ground to a powder. Nutrients from the finely ground almonds are the most available for digestion. The amygdalin in bitter almonds is associated with anti-cancer properties, as is phytate and its breakdown product, inositol.

Almonds are sometimes prepared to be eaten whole, by first soaking them until they begin to sprout, then drying them again. This reduces the phytate content considerably because the sprouting nut generates an enzyme to break down the phytate into inositol and phosphate. These breakdown products are very important nutrients in their own right. Inositol is part of the vitamin B-complex and is needed by every cell in the body, as are adequate amounts of phosphate in the right configuration as it is released from phytate. Other enzymes in the embryo associated with the almond skin break down the starches to sugars. The result of soaking is a deliciously healthful improvement of the almond.

Almonds are mostly fat (55.8 percent) and are also high in protein (21.1 percent). Water is a minor constituent (4.2 percent), as are the digestible carbohydrates—sugar and starch constitute only 6.9 percent. Except for lignin, the fiber (12.9 percent) in almonds is also carbohydrate but contributes very few calories. So, in almonds the ratio of fiber to digestible carbohydrate is very high and they definitely rank as low in carbohydrates, or *low carb,* which means proportionately small amounts of digestible carbohydrates.

Chestnuts

Roasted chestnuts, hot from a brazier, can still be found in European cities. In my own memory, they were sold on city streets in London in the 1940s, and

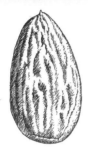

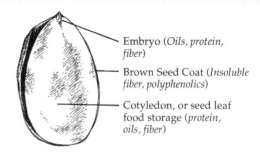

Embryo (*Oils, protein, fiber*)

Brown Seed Coat (*Insoluble fiber, polyphenolics*)

Cotyledon, or seed leaf food storage (*protein, oils, fiber*)

Figure 19.1. Whole Almond   **Figure 19.2.** Open Half Almond

the brazier produced an incredibly welcome aura of warmth and delicious aroma in the midst of the darkness and cold dense fog in late December days. At home we used to roast them over an open fire in a perforated metal tray that was balanced on the red hot coals. This is how the mountain people of Tuscany roast them, and with great effectiveness because they are their staple food for at least a part of the year. During the evening they roast the chestnuts so the shell and skins become completely brittle and can be chipped and broken off to reveal the creamy colored chestnut. This method can be simulated by toasting the chestnuts under a broiler for five minutes or less until the shells are brittle and somewhat charred. This works very well when the chestnuts are fresh and moist, but unfortunately, the same moisture makes chestnuts vulnerable to molds, so if the chestnuts are to be stored, it is better to first dry them. In Tuscany, they are dried over a gently burning fire for two days. A modern food dehydrator set at 140°F successfully achieves the same result in a day. At the end of the drying time, the chestnuts can be easily cracked out of their shells and skins.

The wild chestnut tree (*Castanea sativa*) is native to large areas of Western Europe, and is especially valued in France, Portugal, Spain, and the mountainous regions of Tuscany in Italy. Compared with other tree nuts, chestnuts are remarkably high in starch, and are quite moist due to their high water content. They have a relatively small amount of protein and fat. The nut shell is tough and inedible, as is the skin immediately surrounding the chestnut, which is bitter due to the very high concentration of polyphenolics (tannins) and is usually peeled away. The peeled chestnut still contains considerable amounts of fiber, both soluble and insoluble, spread throughout the starchy bulk of the nut, and antioxidant polyphenolics are present with the fiber. Like all seed foods, chestnuts are also rich in folic acid and other B vitamins, iron, potassium, magnesium and other minerals, and vitamin C.

There are also marrons, which are larger chestnuts that are a cultivated specialty of France and are usually prepared in a sugar syrup as marrons glacées. Fresh chestnuts are inherently very sweet so their presence in desserts need not involve added sugar. Eating chestnuts as a sugary dessert is in sharp contrast to the way chestnuts are eaten as a staple by mountain people, who grind dried chestnuts into flour to make bread, hot cereal, pancakes, polenta, or waffles.

Walnuts

Walnuts contain an abundance of polyunsaturated oils, including the omega–3 oils that are essential for healthy brain and nerve cells, making them a good food for the brain and nervous system. Who can deny that walnuts look like brains inside their shells, and therefore suggest their own value? Historically, the walnut was prized for its oil that was used as an alternative to olive oil in salads. In Eastern Europe especially, a walnut pastry (ideally whole-wheat), which consists of many layers of paper-thin filo dough and plenty of walnuts in the filling, is traditionally made with each new walnut crop. This pastry is almost universally eaten, which ensures that the whole population benefits from the fresh essential oils supplied by the new walnuts.

Among the tree nuts, walnuts stand out as being the richest in polyunsaturated essential oils. All the other common tree nuts, even the related pecans, have monounsaturated oils as their main fat content. Protein is the only other major nutrient in walnuts, supported by fiber, of course, mostly of the insoluble type. Sterols and tocopherols, the fat-soluble antioxidants that protect the reproductive system and prevent oxidative rancidity, are also valuable nutrients supplied along with the polyunsaturated essential oils. Plus, as with all whole-food seeds, walnuts have their fair share of B vitamins and polyphenolic antioxidants.

Other Nuts That Share the Benefits of Almonds and Walnuts

Other nuts, including Brazil nuts, cashew nuts, hazelnuts, macadamia nuts, pecans, pine nuts, and pistachios, also have many of the same benefits as almonds and walnuts. Studies of these nuts have shown they can be part of cholesterol-lowering diets; they have good unsaturated fats, good proteins, and many phytochemicals. And the Brazil nut, with its high selenium content due to the presence of this mineral in the local soil, may have cancer-protective properties as well.

20

What's with Fiber in Oil Seeds?

Somehow people have forgotten how to include enough whole seed foods in their diets. By seed foods, we mean those foods that could grow into a new plant, including grain seeds, beans from leguminous plants, tree nuts, as well as sesame seeds and flaxseeds. They are all highly nutritious simply because they are the beginnings of new plants. Only the grain seeds are well represented in our diet, and even those have had almost all their nutritional advantage removed by being refined into white flours, or being pearled, or polished.

Flax and sesame are examples of oily food-seeds that have an ancient history in our diet and we need these seeds to supply the oils and edible fiber that are rarely found elsewhere in our food crops.

Flaxseed

Flaxseed, also known as linseed, is the oil seed of cooler temperate climates. There is archeological evidence that the ancient Irish and Danish bog people used flaxseed for food and oil, and flax stems for linen fabric. Flaxseed was similarly used by the ancient Greeks and Romans, but flaxseed now seems to be little more than an item in a health food store. Times are changing, however, with the increasing appreciation of the fatty acids in flaxseed oil—the essential fatty acids linoleic (omega-6) acid, and linolenic (omega-3) acid are named after their original source, linseed, after all. Flaxseed is a rich plant source of omega-3 fatty acid that is currently obtained mainly from fish oils. The benefits of these oils are legion, including a healthy heart, reduction of cholesterol especially the harmful LDL cholesterol, and resistance to type-2 diabetes, rheumatoid arthritis, and strokes. By comparison, omega-6 fatty acid is present in such common oils as corn and sunflower, to the exclusion of omega-3 fatty acid oil. Although omega-6 fatty acid is essential, an unbalanced excess can have the adverse effect of causing an increased risk for cancer, diabetes, heart disease, and strokes. Flaxseed oil is 9 percent saturated, 18 percent monounsaturated, and 73 percent polyunsaturated, with 57 percent as omega-3 and only 16 percent as omega-6.

The antioxidant phenolics and tocopherols that preserve the oils of the whole flaxseed are also beneficial. Flaxseed can be kept for at least a year, provided it is stored at a cool temperature and kept dry and away from insect or rodent damage.

The seed of flax is quite small and the hull is edible so the whole seeds are generally eaten in breads, or as a flour made by grinding the seeds without any separation process. The old-fashioned method was with a stone mill, but now flax flour can be made at home in small batches in a high-powered blender. To preserve the oils, it is particularly important to use a cool grinding method. Although it is wise to use newly milled flax flour, it is well-preserved naturally by all the antioxidant phenolics and tocopherols that are also present. According to one experiment, flax flour was not very much changed even after four months at room temperature. At home, we personally make only the amount of flax flour that can be used in a week, and store it in the refrigerator at 40°F. You can easily learn to use a blender to make this flax flour and guarantee yourself a fresh supply.

Sadly, the high concentration of omega-3 fatty acid in old-fashioned flax is seen by some people as a disadvantage. This is because it is so easily oxidized, which makes it difficult to store. But surely it is better to learn to grind your own flax for a fresh supply, than to buy a less beneficial flaxseed that has much smaller amounts of omega-3 fatty acids, as some Canadian manufacturers are doing.

The rich supply of omega-3 fatty acid is, after all, the main reason to be eating flaxseed. Linseed is usually a dark brown color and typically contains 50–60 percent omega-3 acid in the oil. But the omega-3 reduced variety from Canada has only a meager 5 percent of the omega-3 left in. This variety, called solin seed, can be recognized by its golden color, but it is supposedly available only to the commercial cooking oil producers and hopefully can be avoided by consumers. *Note:* In the United States, a different yellow-colored flaxseed, called Omega, has been developed, and this has just as much omega-3 fatty acid in it as the brown seeded flax. The Flaxseed Council of Canada insists that all their varieties—both brown and golden—were all developed using traditional methods and do not contain GMO's (genetically modified organisms), which leads me to presume that their flax contains no non-flax genes, only those that occur naturally in flax, but it is too easy for plant growers to play havoc with nutrients, and too difficult to remain vigilant and selective of all foods. This makes it immensely important to use research to discover the attributes a food plant already has, before deciding to modify them to suit the whims of commercial production and marketing strategy.

The Soluble Fiber and Lignans in Flaxseed

The fiber associated with flaxseed is especially valuable in that it consists of an unusually high proportion of soluble fiber. No other common seed food has so much, and researchers, including David Jenkins in Toronto, attribute at least part of the cholesterol-reducing effect of whole flax to this soluble fiber. Even more important is that the oxidized cholesterol in the LDLs is selectively reduced. When flaxseed is soaked, it immediately becomes gummy due to the soluble fiber in the edible hull. The insoluble fraction contains substantial amounts of the large polyphenolic lignin, associated with cellulose, and lignans, which are much smaller phenolic polymers than lignin itself and much more readily absorbed when eaten. These lignans have pronounced anti-cancer effects, and should be an indispensable part of any diet. Lignans seem to give significant protection against breast and prostate cancers. The color of the seed is due to another group of antioxidant compounds (flavonoids) that are active anti-inflammatory agents. Dark-colored flaxseed most likely contains more of these substances, which makes it preferable to light golden-colored flax.

Other nutrients of note in the whole flaxseed are the minerals calcium, magnesium, phosphorus, and potassium. The digestible carbohydrate content of flaxseeds is barely detectable because fiber, oil, and protein make up the bulk of the flaxseed. The protein in flaxseeds is similar to the essential amino acids in soybeans and, as such, is a valuable complement to the proteins of grains, such as wheat. Flaxseed flour combined with wheat in bread makes an especially nutritious combination, with enhanced protein, fat, and fiber qualities.

Sesame

Sesame is the oil seed of China, Egypt, India, Japan, Mesopotamia, North Africa, Persia, Turkey, and all the tropics and subtropics. My first experience with sesame was halvah, and I considered my mother very adventurous for bringing it home in the 1950s. At that time, England was still reeling from the shortages caused by the Second World War, and we felt fortunate if we could buy just good basic food. Halvah, made from sesame seeds and honey, came from the eastern Mediterranean and was to us a very exotically flavored sweet.

Sesame has a curious, nutty, but also somewhat smoky, flavor that perfectly complements the flavor of wheat bread. Just as they do in the Middle East, you can sprinkle sesame seeds on sandwich buns or cracker breads, and that will enhance the nutritional value of the breads.

The sesame contains a high proportion of oil and can be ground to a paste, known as tahini, that is similar in texture to almond butter or smooth peanut butter. Whole-seed tahini is superb and shows it is not necessary to remove the hulls in order to make a good tahini. Nor is there any need to remove the hulls before sprinkling the seeds on breads. Most varieties of sesame are white, so the sesame-tahini color is the same whether the hulls are removed or not. Black varieties are mostly Japanese and are used for the production of sesame oil.

Sesame oil is frequently used in Asian salads and cooking, giving off a flavor that seems quintessentially Asian. The extraordinary stability of the oil is due to the generous amount of phenolic antioxidants, vitamin E, and related compounds that are concentrated in the oil. The oil is valuable as a rich source of unsaturated fatty acids, particularly the essential fatty acids.

The edible fiber in the seed hull is associated with minerals, especially calcium. Phytate and oxalate are also present in the hull, and they are disadvantageous because they will bind metals too strongly to be easily digested. However, phytate has the redeeming characteristics of combating cancer, especially colon cancer, and being a source of inositol. Except for about a quarter of the total fiber, which is soluble, the hull fiber is mostly insoluble.

Other Oil Seeds

Around the world there are other seeds, such as pumpkin, squash, and sunflower seeds, that are rich in good oils and have been used as a basic part of the diet for centuries. And in Chapter 22 you will find additional seeds that are all great sources of good oils, phytochemicals, including vitamin E and proteins.

21

What's with Fiber in Fruits?

Protective Power in Fruits

Fruit is the ultimate reward from the plant kingdom, and is the perfect dessert, sweet and dramatically colored and flavored. The variety is superb: Apples, berries, citrus, dates, figs, grapes, melons, peaches, pears, plums, raspberries, strawberries, tropical fruits, and many more. Moreover, the reward is more than the sweet, sugary taste because all fruits have vitamin C and antioxidant phytochemicals that are incredibly protective against disease. The whole fruit has the power to regulate the way all that sugar enters the system. Under its influence, the sugar is released into the bloodstream gradually and gently, and not too much at once, which prevents a sudden drop in blood sugar caused by too much insulin released too fast. Fiber and antioxidant phytochemicals are given the most credit for this controlling effect, but fruits also contain significant amounts of B vitamins, which are essential to the efficient release of energy from sugars. In addition, the naturally high ratio of potassium to sodium in fruits contributes to a natural control of blood pressure. There are also, no doubt, other, not yet isolated, compounds in fruits, that help to assimilate all that sugar in such a controlled manner. At least part of the reason that fruit fiber can restrain the release of sugar is simply because the sugar is trapped in the fiber network as it is carried through the digestive system.

An abundance of fruit should be considered an essential part of the diet, and not just something to take when you visit people, or buy as a Saturday treat. Fortunately, there is a tendency to feast on fruits while they are in season and at the peak of their perfection. This is all right because fruits have a very high water content, from 75 percent for bananas to 86 percent for oranges. Roger Troy Wilson, who wrote *Let's Do Lunch,* found he could overcome his near-lifelong obesity and lose weight by eating only fruit for desserts and snacks. He actually ate a wide enough range of foods to feel satisfied, but made sure he avoided the high-fat processed foods, and those made from refined flour and sugar. Whenever he had a craving for a disastrously fattening food away from home, he ate raisins, which he kept with him all the time.

Grapes, and peaches, pears, plums, and other fruits with pits are eaten fresh or dried, and their nutritional value changes from fresh to dried. The drying process is akin to cooking and there is a release of nutrients, including polyphenolics, from the fibrous cells that have burst open and softened as the water evaporated. The concentrating effect and the release of nutrients from the fibrous cells gives dried fruit an increased antioxidant effect, weight for weight, over fresh fruit—the antioxidant effect of *dried* fruit is comparable to, or exceeds, that seen for whole grains.

If fruit is cooked at all, only a little water, just enough to allow for evaporation, is used, since the fruit itself is so water-laden. Seedy fruit, such as raspberries, strawberries, or grapes with seeds and tough skin especially benefit from cooking because the boiling process releases nutrients into the juice from the seeds and skins that cannot be easily released by our digestive system. Removing the skins and seeds by straining the fruit after cooking, results in highly nutritious liquid concentrates that often surpass the original fruit in both flavor and benefit. Berry concentrates are delicious with fresh plain yogurt. Fresh fruit is so rich in nutrients that it is a pity to remove the fiber residue during juicing. Blenders that purée the fresh fruit and preserve all the components are preferable to juicers that remove all the fiber and associated compounds, leaving only the juice.

Precious Pectin in Fruits

As with all plant parts, fruits are built from microscopic cells, and fruit cells have their own special characteristics. The fruit cell walls are generally similar to all other plant cell walls, with soft pectin, and sometimes lignin, surrounding the firmer structural cellulose. Pectin is a soluble fiber and a carbohydrate that cannot be digested until it reaches the bacteria of the colon, where it produces short-chain fatty acids. These short-chain fatty acids include propionic and butyric acids, which are also naturally present in some bacterially fermented cheeses, and acetic acid, which is found in vinegar. These acids are easily absorbed and lead to favorable HDL in the blood. The calories delivered to the body from soluble fiber via these short-chain fatty acids are only half those that come from a corresponding amount of digestible carbohydrates, such as sugar or starch.

Insoluble cellulose fiber is a glucose polymer and, therefore, also a carbohydrate. But its structure prevents it from being digested, even by the bacteria of the colon, and it usually passes through the body without producing any substance that would be absorbed and generate calories. Its value is in its ability to swell by absorbing plenty of water and carry food through our entire digestive system. Cellulose gives necessary bulk to stools. Some bulking also occurs due to the increased growth in beneficial bacteria when there is plenty of pectin reaching the colon. Fruit is often credited with facilitating bowel movements, but pectin is given medicinally to reduce diarrhea by encouraging the growth of friendly bacteria. There are other compounds present in some fruits, such as figs, prunes, and raisins, that have an effect on bowel movement beyond the mere presence of pectin. A balanced, friendly bacterial population is essential to everyone's health and must be maintained by introducing friendly bacteria through foods, such as yogurt, and then encouraging their growth with soluble fiber from whole-plant foods.

There has definitely been a conspiracy between fruit and our ancestors with a great desire for sweet foods. Over the centuries, they selected the sweetest, most beautifully colored, and most interestingly flavored fruits, and the seeds of those fruits became the future generations of fruit plants. There have been many genetic manipulations, such as grafting and crossing, to achieve the fruits of today. In the future, this selective process should also include the most nutritious fruits.

The Sugars in Fruit

Fruit sugar is usually a mixture of glucose and fructose, and rarely sucrose, which is identical with cane sugar. When digested separately from fruit, glucose assimilation is faster than that of fructose or sucrose, which emphasizes how effective whole fruit is in slowing down sugar absorption to a level that is kind to the body. The B vitamins are well represented in all fruits, which allows the sugars inside the cells of the plant to be properly used.

The miraculous processes that take place in each cell of living material, especially when there is a plentiful supply of glucose and fructose, are worthy of attention. Very often, plants can manufacture compounds that people cannot. The compounds that promote the controlled release of energy are to be respected, and it is no longer justifiable to discard them, and their fiber, as useless. The old days of thinking that only proteins, fats, and carbohydrates were needed to survive are gone. If these are eaten without any of the controlling compounds in plant cells, your body would not be able to process them in a fully beneficial way. It is now obvious that the current long-term deficit of whole-plant foods has lead to such diseases as diabetes and, especially, coronary artery disease.

Fruits to the Rescue for British Sailors

Vitamin C and various antioxidant polyphenolics are among the components of fruit found to be so beneficial. Scurvy was the first condition to be recognized as a deficiency disease, but even though it was realized that citrus fruits effectively alleviated the symptoms of the deficiency, it took 200 years to recognize that scurvy was specifically caused by a lack of vitamin C in the diet. When fruits and vegetables were not sufficiently supplied to sailors or overland travelers, its symptoms were noted: bleeding gums, bruises, painful joints, skin hemorrhages, and eventually, death. But as soon as vitamin C, in the form of fruits, was ingested in adequate amounts, these symptoms disappeared.

Phenolic Compounds Protect Vitamin C

The colored substances in fruits are antioxidant polyphenolics, and these work with vitamin C to stabilize, enhance, and prolong its activity. But it has only been in the last decade that the tannins and the flavor and color compounds in fruit have been valued for their phenomenally important roles in human health. In 1935, Albert Szent-Györgyi observed that blood vessels were greatly strengthened by including *whole* red peppers and *whole* lemon juice in the diet, rather than pure vitamin C alone, but the significance of his observations have been neglected until now. They are, however, immensely important to the person with diabetes who experiences the effects of weakened blood vessels in blindness due to macular degeneration, or impaired circulation that can lead to amputations. The early signs of diabetes can often be alleviated and the disease halted when the diet includes abundant whole-plant foods, with their accompanying antioxidant polyphenolics.

Vitamin C is also known to be necessary for the healthy maintenance and regeneration of collagen tissue in the joints. The colored polyphenolics seem to enhance the properties of vitamin C that maintain healthy joints and reduce vulnerability to arthritis. And research has shown that rheumatoid arthritis is diminished when there are sufficient polyphenolics in the diet, including naturally occurring salicylic acid (aspirin), which is anti-inflammatory. These polyphenolic color and flavor compounds from whole-plant foods have been found to be active in preventing, or at least reducing, the impact of cancer, cardiovascular disease, and diabetes. In fact, both colored and colorless polyphenolics have been found valuable in preventing these conditions. A healthier and happier life is to be gained by eating plant foods only in their whole form, and, since carbohydrate foods are essentially of plant origin, this means eating all carbohydrates in the whole-plant form.

Where are these beneficial polyphenolics concentrated? They exist wherever the color or flavor of the fruit is the most intense, usually in the skin, and sometimes around the seeds. Their activity in the fruits is protective. They link easily with proteins and carbohydrates so they are ready for healing action at the site of injury to a fruit. Lignin is part of the strengthening fiber in some cells and is made from carbohydrate units linked to phenolics (*see* Chapter 1). A darkened color on a cut fruit reveals its ability to rapidly absorb oxygen from the air and turn it into a brown oxidized substance that protects the cells beneath. It's interesting to realize that these same compounds are healing for people too, and that their function is related to their ability to link so easily with carbohydrates, proteins, and oxygen.

All this makes fruits valuable, not just for their vitamin C content, but for their antioxidant power. Previously, citrus fruit, kiwis, and red peppers were valued simply because they were the highest in vitamin C; now some of the fruits that are low in vitamin C are also recognized as worthy because they contain such a rich supply of polyphenolics. Blueberries, grapes, pomegranates, and strawberries are being given far more praise for being healthy than ever before.

Apples

There is now an explanation for the old saying that an apple a day keeps the doctor away. The healthfulness of apples, and the reason for the old saying, comes in how apples supply soluble fiber, which aids in maintaining a healthy cholesterol level, as well as in their antioxidant power from the polyphenolics they contain. The skin is richest in the colored antioxidants, but other active antioxidants are distributed throughout the apple. The value of apples also lies in their year-round availability. They store so well, it's easy to eat an apple a day for most of the year.

Even though they contain only small amounts of vitamin C, apples have a generous amount of pectin soluble fiber that can be used to make jam with other fruits, such as strawberries. The sweetness indicates there are plenty of sugars present, mostly fructose, with some glucose. Apples illustrate the beneficial effect of the whole fruit on the speed with which the sugars are assimilated. They can be eaten whole, bite by bite, they can be cooked into an apple sauce, or they can be prepared as a clear juice. In each case, the sugars are eaten in the same quantity, but as juice the sugars enter the bloodstream much more rapidly because it is devoid of the apple fiber, most of the B vitamins, and anything else that would moderate the sugary jolt. The apple eaten whole is not only eaten slowly, but the chunks of apple will not easily release their sugar content. When they do, all the necessary compounds are right there accompanying them to produce a gently sustained release into the bloodstream, and an easy uptake by all of the needy body cells.

Apricots

The Hunzas in Pakistan's mountainous Hunza Valley have a reputation for leading long, healthy, active lives, and one of their main subsistence foods, besides yogurt, is apricots. They grow large quantities of them, which they eat in both sweet and savory dishes, as well as in their 100-percent whole wheat breads.

Fresh apricots are delicious, but dried apricots develop a wonderful flavor and character of their own and can be easily stored for a constant year-round supply. The sweetness of dried apricots is perhaps reduced by the polyphenolics' binding of the sugar released from the cell walls during drying, and the tartness they acquire is due to the malic acid present. This acid is also in plums to about the same extent, and probably explains the laxative properties of both fruits because malic acid behaves like dietary fiber. Malic acid is not digested until it reaches the bacteria of the colon.

The color and flavor of apricots are due to an abundance of antioxidant polyphenolics, including anthocyanins, carotenes, and lutein, which are less often produced in fruit. The carotenes and lutein are especially valuable in preserving eyesight because they protect the retina from macular degeneration. Apricots supply only a small amount of vitamin C, but its effect is stabilized by the presence of the powerful antioxidant polyphenolics. Apricots are particularly protective against cancer and cardiovascular disease.

Bananas

Bananas are moderately high in vitamin C and are uncolored, yet they still have good value as fruit. Although their fiber is associated with a colorless form of antioxidant polyphenolics, these give the banana an antioxidant rating almost as high as a grapefruit and even higher than an apple. Bananas have significant amounts of starch and sucrose, as well as glucose and fructose, fiber, and suitable quantities of B vitamins. Another benefit comes from their particularly high potassium-to-sodium ratio, which aids in maintaining a healthy blood pressure. Bananas are among the known natural suppliers of inulin and related fructooligosaccharides (FOS). These, in turn, are undigested until they reach the colon, but they have great value because they encourage the proliferation of the bifidobacteria in the colon, which are among the healthiest colonic bacteria known to date. The bifidobacteria digest the FOS and produce acetic acid, which makes the colon healthily acidic. When the acetic acid is absorbed, it acts to moderate cholesterol levels. Bulkier stools, another result of the increased bacterial quantity, provide increased immunity and relief from constipation.

Blackberries

The wild blackberry is widely distributed in temperate and Nordic climates, and is a wonderful resource in hard times. I know this from my own childhood in London during World War II. In the midst of food rationing and all the chaos produced by bombings, we took all the bowls we possessed and went out to Hayes Common, where we picked pounds and pounds of ripe, fragrant blackberries. My father made these into blackberry jelly and we feasted for weeks afterwards.

In Scandinavia, the berries of summer are boiled into a juice and stored for use in winter desserts. Blackberries are worth preserving, especially as a juice concentrate. They are tremendously rich in the colored anthocyanins (antioxidant polyphenolics). When blackberries were tested for their total antioxidant power, they had a value of 2,036 for their *oxygen radical absorbance capacity* (ORAC). Only blueberries scored higher (2,400 ORAC) among the fresh fruits. Boiling the fruit with water seems to facilitate the extraction of these compounds into the juice—they are very heat stable. The entire fruit—skins, seeds, and pulp—is extracted during the boiling, which is usually just long enough to make the seeds separate easily when the mixture is strained. Only the seeds, remnants of the pulp, and skin of the blackberries are kept in the strainer and discarded. The collected juice contains fiber and all the fruit-cell extractables, such as folate and potassium, as well as the highly colored anthocyanins and many other polyphenolics, and it is very healthful.

Blueberries

Blueberries in the United States, bilberries in northern Europe, whortleberries in Russia, and huckleberries in the western United States, are all *vaccinium* species and all are closely related botanically. The reputation of English bilberry jam to help reduce the effects of glare, especially after dark, can also be applied to American blueberries and huckleberries. Bilberries are often collected in the wild rather than cultivated, and are generally smaller than blueberries, which seems to give bilberries the highest values for antioxidant power and concentration of anthocyanins among the *vaccinium* species.

Bilberries already had a reputation for healing well before we were awakened to the French paradox and the recognition of the healing powers of fruit polyphenolics. There is even a French pharmaceutical product that contains fermented bilberry juice and is a particularly rich source of bilberry's polyphenolic compounds. It is prescribed for its blood-vessel-strengthening properties. Perhaps the polyphenolics from the bilberry prescription, as well as those from wine grapes, are responsible for the paradoxically low rate of cardiovascular disease among the French.

More recently, Jim Joseph, a researcher at Tufts University, has discovered the effect of blueberries on the brains of rats. When the diet contained blueberries, both memory and coordination were remarkably improved in the rats he studied. A similar effect was produced from strawberries and spinach.

Cantaloupe

As you might imagine from its glorious orange color, the cantaloupe is rich in beta-carotenes, from which the body can produce vitamin A. These beta-carotenes also have antioxidant activity that protects against cancer. They have the advantage of being fat soluble, so they can protect a different part of cells than the more water-soluble antioxidant polyphenolics. The polyphenolics in melons have not been studied very much, but flavorful and anti-inflammatory salicylic-acid derivatives have been found in them. Salicylic acid acetate is a phenolic compound widely known as aspirin. Various compounds related to salicylic acid have been found in fruit, and they have similiar anti-inflammatory effects as pharmaceutical aspirin. But the advantage of salicylic-acid derivatives in fruit are that they are diluted by the fiber and do not cause damage to the stomach lining.

The plant cell fiber, the sugars, the B vitamins, potassium, and other plant cell materials are all there in well-ripened melons, which are a thirst-quenching, refreshing treasure among the summer fruits, especially because they provide antioxidants that protect the cornea and retina of the eyes, and the skin, against the sun.

Cherries

Even though the cherry season is short, people tend to eat as many as possible during that time, which is a great benefit because cherries have a remarkably cleansing effect on the digestive system. Cherry juice is now prepared commercially, and is a way of preserving the flavor and benefits of cherries into the winter months. The most nutritious cherry juice includes all the fiber, soluble skin, and seed components. In cherries, along with the expected pectin and cellulose fiber, there is sorbitol, which has a theoretical energy value similar to cane sugar, but delivers far fewer calories. Sorbitol tastes sweet, but is not a carbohydrate (though very similar), and it is quite laxative and diuretic. Since only a small proportion of sorbitol enters the blood to supply energy, it is often added to prepared low-calorie foods, and can be used as a sweetener for anyone with diabetes.

Cherries are much valued in folk medicine and there are some interesting anecdotal cures worth mentioning, including their beneficial effect on both osteo- and rheumatoid arthritis, and particularly on gout, a related condition. People who have been helped by cherry juice say they drink at least a cup of black cherry juice each day. It makes sense that the polyphenolic antioxidants in cherries work with vitamin C to help repair or maintain the collagen in joints, offering some logic to the anecdotal improvements and cures. Even though, to my knowledge, the scientific journals have not yet reported on this, it is possible that the combination of polyphenolics, sorbitol, and benzoic-acid derivatives in cherries are responsible for the reported diuretic properties and benefits to people with gout or gouty arthritis.

A bark extract from the wild black-cherry tree of the northeastern United States was used by Native Americans as a cough medicine, and its use was continued by the early settlers from Europe. Similar usefulness can probably be found in the fruit of this wild black-cherry tree.

Citrus Fruit

Oranges, lemons, grapefruit, and limes are the famous vitamin-C-rich fruits that prevent the deficiency disease of scurvy because these citrus fruits contain more vitamin C than any other, with the possible exception of the kiwi and the strawberry. In the 1770s, twenty years after the naval British surgeon James Lind made his 1753 observations about vitamin C preventing scurvy, Captain James Cook became the first to demonstrate that long sea voyages could be undertaken without the crew becoming sick from scurvy by taking particular care to provide plenty of fresh fruits and vegetables, especially oranges and lemons, during his voyage around the world.

This was not the end of scurvy, however. In 1849, many of the goldrush miners arriving in California by land and sea had scurvy. Babies, too, became susceptible to the disease when artificial milks were prepared for them in the 1880s and 1890s. At that time, proteins, fats, and carbohydrates seemed to define all food, a prize example of how people in the past decided they knew enough to make a purified food that would be nutritionally sufficient. Historical examples such as these should cause people to be extremely wary of purifying or synthesizing foods, which could be excluding valuable, even essential, nutrients not yet fully understood. It was not until 1932 that C. G. King, among others in the United States, and Albert Szent-Györgyi in Hungary all independently published their results on the isolation of vitamin C and its ability to prevent scurvy, studies for which Dr. Szent-Györgyi received the Nobel Prize.

With their fiber, citrus fruits have much more to offer than vitamin C alone. Gone are the days when just one or two compounds were given credit for a healthy attribute. Today, it is generally acknowledged that all components of foods, especially plant foods, work in concert. The bioflavonoids in citrus fruits are a good example because the polyphenolic compounds in them preserve and enhance the activity of vitamin C. Eating oranges boosts immunity from infections, protects from cardiovascular disease, and has anti-cancer activity, and this can all be connected to the orange's combination of vitamin C and polyphenolics. Oranges in generous amounts also provide protection from strokes as a result of their high concentration of potassium, which moderates blood pressure. A meaningful amount of folate is also ingested when generous amounts of oranges are eaten. Folate, a B vitamin, has just recently been given high priority in the diet when it was finally added to refined flour in the late 1990s to compensate for the missing folate from wheat germ. Besides being a crucial vitamin for pregnant women, to avoid the possibility of spina bifida or other neural-tube defects in newborn babies, folate is now given credit for reducing homocysteine levels in the blood, and consequently reducing susceptibilty to Alzheimer's disease, diabetes, and cardiovascular disease. In addition, oranges contain significant amounts of lutein and beta-carotene and are considered a good fruit for eye health, especially in aging. And, in her book, *Miracle Cures,* Jean Carper writes about grapefruit fiber pectin and its use as a supplement for lowering cholesterol.

The peel of oranges is routinely discarded, but this is a pity because the peel is an immensely rich source of orange oils and the soluble-fiber pectin,

Skin Defense

An interesting effect of eating citrus peel is its benefit as a skin tonic—it has an anecdotal reputation for helping to prevent and cure acne. In connection with this, the known first line of defense against acne is to never wash the skin with hard water and soap, which leave a residue that is very hard to wash off and can cause blocked pores, especially in teenage skin. Soft water and distilled water are preferable because they are compatible with soap and give a rich soluble lather. Soap can be avoided altogether, if desired, by washing with a moisturizing lotion.

and the peel of oranges can be delicious. Homemade orange marmalade—whole oranges grated in a food processor, cooked in water, and then sweetened with a little honey—is a magnificent condiment. Since it is homemade, we add it generously to yogurt as a dessert, eat it with cereals at breakfast and, of course, spread it on bread. In fruit breads and cakes, it is a delicious substitute for candied peel. Marmalades can be lemon, lime, and grapefruit-based as well, but the orange has a sweetness that mellows their flavor.

Another way to eat the peel of oranges and lemons is in smoothies, fresh fruit mixes that can be made in a blender. In a study done at our Center, we saw for ourselves that blueberries, grapes, oranges with their peel, pineapple, and strawberries made into a smoothie increased blood levels of antioxidants within thirty minutes of drinking the delicious concoction. Also, orange juice produced by crushing the whole fruit will include some of the oils from the skin. One caution, however: When any citrus peel is to be eaten, it is important to use fruit known to be free of toxic pesticides.

Cranberries

Cranberries are a magnificent crimson red, and have a distinctly tart flavor. Historically native to North America, they are relished as an accompaniment to turkey. An old American food, pemmican, was originally a dried mixture of cranberries with venison. It carried Native Americans through the winter in good health, and early settlers and explorers who copied their diet felt the advantages too, evidently not discouraged by the tartness—perhaps they believed it was good for them.

Cranberries are rich in vitamin C and polyphenolic antioxidants. And cranberries have a large amount of benzoic acid, closely related to the polyphenolics—its presence explains the diuretic effect of cranberries. Their effect in preventing urinary tract infections has recently been explained as being due to some of the more complex polyphenolics they contain. These polyphenolics are thought to coat the urinary tract and prevent unwanted bacteria from adhering to it, so infection cannot occur. The same is true for stomach-ulcer bacteria—the presence of cranberries prevents them from adhering to the stomach lining. Cranberries also have anti-cancer activity and promote good cardiovascular health.

Since cranberries have seeds just big enough to be a bother, and have exceedingly tough skins, they are best prepared as a juice. Boil them for about thirty minutes, until the berries burst and soften, and then strain them to retrieve almost all the soft soluble fiber and juice, leaving the skins and seeds behind. After this process, the skins are almost colorless—the boiling probably extracts the color and the compounds from the seeds and brings them into the juice, making them more available for digestion than they might have been in the raw, whole cranberries. The soluble-fiber pulp that is collected with the juice acts as a natural thickener, and if it is sufficiently concentrated, the juice will set like a jelly.

Dates

Watching dates ripen on the stem after they have been picked is quite a revelation. They change from dry pale yellow to juicy dark brown in just a few days when left in a bowl in a warm room. Once again it was the local (Palo Alto) farmers' market that made this experience possible; there they were, a display of at least four distinctly different kinds of fresh dates *(Phoenix dactylifera)* that had been grown in the Coachella Valley of the southern California desert.

The Sacred Fruit of the Arabs

The largest date plantations are in Saudi Arabia, which is appropriate because dates were considered the sacred food of the Arabs, and the date is a staple food in the desert regions of the Middle East and North Africa. For long periods at a time, desert-nomad Arabs eat only dates and camel milk and remain very healthy. Dried dates still contain a little water (15 percent), as do other dried fruits, and can be stored for a year or more in this state. When dried even further, they lose their juiciness completely, become hard, and can then be ground into a flour. The date sugar found in grocery stores is actually *whole* date flour. It contains everything originally in the date flesh, except water, and the dates can be stored indefinitely in the form of this flour. As with most natural foods, dates also come packaged, so if you want natural dates, be sure to notice whether any other ingredients have been added.

The sugar content of dried dates is high (68 percent), which is to be expected from their sweet flavor, but surprisingly this is comparable with other dried fruits, such as raisins (69 percent). The sugar in dates is mostly a mixture of glucose and fructose, with glucose only slightly higher than fructose.

Dates contain plenty of antioxidant polyphenolics, recognizable by the rich reddish-brown coloring. In fact, dates have a series of these compounds named especially for them, so if dates are ever found to have special health attributes, these will likely be the reason. As it is, there is a plethora of polyphenolics present to make dates a natural way to prevent cardiovascular disease and reduce the risk of cancer and diabetes. These compounds are linked with most of the sugars and the fiber, and are the reason why the sugars from dates digest more slowly than refined cane sugar.

Dates are particularly rich in the B-vitamin niacin and its precursors, as well as other B vitamins, such as pantothenic acid and B$_6$, all of which are essential for the healthy assimilation of the sugars in dates. These B vitamins and the high quantity of potassium and other minerals, such as iron and magnesium, are fairly evenly distributed throughout the fleshy part of the date.

In fresh dates, vitamin C is also present in amounts similar to other fresh fruits, such as cherries, but it disappears from dried dates. We have a theory, however, that perhaps the vitamin C becomes bound to the polyphenolics and only *looks* as though it has disappeared. After all, the Arab nomads don't suffer from scurvy on their limited diet of dates and camel milk. As with vitamin C, carotenes are also found in quantities similar to cherries and other fruits.

Date fiber is the cell wall material that is spread throughout the date, enclosing everything else. It is composed mostly of insoluble cellulose and soluble pectin, but also contains more appreciable amounts of lignin than other fruits. Basically, the components of whole dates are not remarkably different from those of other fruits, and dates, with their brown, gooey appearance, provide well-rounded fruit nutrition.

Figs

The first time I was given a fresh, green Calmyrna fig at peak ripeness, I was well into my twenties. We were in a Greek garden when our host picked the most delicious fig I have ever eaten, and none since have ever surpassed that thrilling sweetness.

The two kinds of figs with which I am most familiar, green Calmyrna and black mission, are both delicate to handle. Attempting to have them arrive in stores in prime condition is almost impossible because to be perfectly flavored they also must be very soft and juicy. Soft and juicy figs are prone to molds, and if these take hold, the flavor becomes awful, which is probably one reason why some people dislike figs.

Before they can mold, therefore, figs should be dried, and if the flavor is off, it's best to discard them. Good figs have a wonderful, sweet flavor when properly dried, without any additives, and this is the way they are usually sold.

In Mediterranean countries where figs easily grow to perfection, they have been the poor man's staple food for millennia, an indication of their importance in the healthful Mediterranean diet. Figs have an unusual structure for a fruit. They consist of over a thousand miniature fruits, each with its own seed. Figs have an abundance of fiber, mostly insoluble, but meaningful amounts of soluble fiber are also present.

Dried figs are concentrated sources of nutrients, which compare well with other fruits. Fructose and glucose sugars are in approximately equal amounts, and there is very little sucrose. There are significant amounts of protein and oil, mostly derived from the seeds, and figs appear to have more calcium, copper, iron, potassium, zinc, and vitamins B_1 (thiamine), B_6, and pantothenic acid than other dried fruits.

The laxative and diuretic properties of figs are well known. The medicinal form is syrup, obtained by boiling the figs, straining them to remove the seeds and then concentrating the extract, which would contain the seed extract—it may well be that the diuretic and laxative quality of the syrup is supplied by the seeds. Figs have not been studied to speak of, so there is much still to be to learned about them, which could help to explain these properties. So far, the purple skins of figs have been recognized as a good source of colored antioxidant polyphenolics (anthocyanins) of the kind known to enhance the properties of vitamin C in maintaining healthy joints. Figs, in general, contain a number of other polyphenolics that are valuable in reducing cancer, cardiovascular disease, and diabetes.

Grapes and Raisins

Grapes have an incredible reputation for promoting good health. For centuries, in many Mediterranean countries, after the grape harvest in early fall the *grape cure* has been recommended as a means of treating chronic bowel disorders which means eating only grapes for one or two days. According to J. H. Kellogg, writing his book *Colon Hygiene* in 1927, the effectiveness is partly due to the generous amount of tartaric acid in grapes. Grapes are also the world's largest fruit crop, and because they are the basis of wine, they have probably been studied more than any other fruit.

Grapes have a great variety and abundance of polyphenolics, including the brilliantly colored anthocyanins that are mostly found in dark grape skins. The seeds have also yielded enough polyphenolics to warrant selling grape-seed extract as a health food supplement. The general effect of these antioxidants is disease prevention, especially against cancer, cardiovascular disease, and diabetes.

The dried grape, better known as the raisin, is also replete with these same compounds, but in the drying process some compounds tend to be bound by the fiber matrix. In the body, they are released during the bacterial digestion of soluble fiber in the colon and are absorbed along with the short-chain fatty acids that are simultaneously released. The raisin is the stable storage form of the grape and has been recognized as particularly appropriate for athletes. In one of the studies at our own center, triathletes competing in a vigorous swim, a bicycle ride, and a run ate raisins as a sustaining snack at intervals during the competition. Their blood glucose level was maintained in a steady state, and the antioxidants protected vulnerable cells from DNA damage. This latter activity is immediate evidence of the protection given by the antioxidants in grapes (and other fruits) against cancer. In another study, also in our center, antioxidant levels in the blood rose rapidly after eating raisins.

Grapes and raisins have laxative effects that can be attributed to the tartaric acid they contain. Tartaric acid is unusual in fruit. Apart from grapes, only the tamarind has been found to contain substantial amounts of this acid. (The tamarind tree is grown in tropical and subtropical Africa, India, and Southeast Asia.) Tamarind's reputation as a laxative is similar to that of raisins, but more specifically, tamarind has the reputation of promoting bile excretion. Both of these attributes have now been investigated for raisins. Bile-acid excretion has been shown to rise, as has the bulk and acidity of stools, when a handful of raisins are eaten twice daily. The bulked stools aid regular and comfortable elimination and a reduced transit time of only one or two days. The increased bile-acid excretion demonstrates the fast removal of bile acids from the colon. This, along with the increased acidity in the colon when raisins are regularly eaten, encourages a healthy colonic microflora and the prevention of colon cancer. Raisins are also a particularly concentrated source of potassium, which helps to naturally maintain a healthy blood pressure.

Kiwi

Oil of wintergreen has a wonderfully healing fragrance due to natural methyl salicylate, and it's often used in ointments to ease the sting from cuts and scrapes. For me, it's a smell reminiscent of childhood and the school playground. Kiwis have the same fragrance, only milder and tempered with other fruity flavors. Salicylates, related to anti-inflammatory aspirin, belong to the large group of compounds known as phenolics, which have been identified in several fruits besides kiwis, including cantaloupes, grapes, grapefruits, and raspberries. Kiwis ripen here in California during the winter and provide an exotic addition to the apples, bananas, oranges, and pears available then.

The kiwi's origin in China explains its earlier name of Chinese gooseberry. By the 1950s, New Zealand was growing kiwis in quantity and exporting them. Their skin is curiously furry and tough, their seeds are small and beautifully arranged in the center of the fruit, and, except for the tough skin, the whole fruit can be eaten raw. The vitamin-C content of kiwis is extraordinarily high, on a par with lemons. Additionally, kiwis supply plenty of potassium and fiber, both soluble and insoluble, some simple sugars in the form of glucose and fructose, and adequate mounts of the B vitamins and beta-carotene.

Mango

The large seed in the center of the mango is covered with long stringy fiber that is easily described as insoluble. Surrounding the pit and the stringy fiber is an incredibly delicious and juicy fruit pulp, but the skin is usually too tough to consider eating. Mangoes contain more sucrose than either glucose or fructose, which suggests they may also contain more oligosaccharides than are generally found in fruits and vegetables.

As expected for fruits, mangoes contain a generous amount of vitamin C, plenty of potassium, and very little sodium. The intense yellow of the mango is due to an exceptionally high concentration of beta-carotene that is three times greater than in a fresh apricot.

Mangoes are a tropical fruit originating in India, and grown throughout Southeast Asia and other tropical climates. They are eaten both fresh and dried, and are also made into pickles and chutney. My mouth waters at the mere thought of mango chutney, but I have never tasted pickled mango here or growing up in Britain. Mangoes are normally picked firm, and are not tree-ripened.

Unripe mangoes are pickled, and also made into vinegar. In the Philippines, a very small mango is brined and pickled much the same as olives, and is valued as a pasta sauce ingredient. The pickling process involves soaking the cut fruit in brine for four to five weeks, during which time there is a buildup of lactic bacteria. Eaten at this stage, the pickles would provide valuable lactic bacteria for the digestive system, as well as lactic acid and acetic acid (vinegar acid) and B vitamins. The bacteria ferment a portion of the dietary fiber, most likely the simplest sugars and pectins, and leave behind the cellulose. Commercially, the pickles are usually further treated with sugar and vinegar and then pasteurized and packaged for sale.

Peaches

The arrival of peaches in the markets coincides with the full heat of summer, and this is one of the most protective fruits against the ravages of strong sunlight on the skin, and the effects of vigorous exercise. Peaches are fairly rich in beta-carotenes, which tend to concentrate in the skin and give antioxidant protection against sunburn. Antioxidant polyphenolics, including the colored pigments inside the peach around the peach pit, as well as in the peach skin, are even more abundantly present. These polyphenolics add to the beneficial effects of peach juice applied to the skin, and also contribute to the wonderfully refreshing fragrance of peaches and their juice. Alpha-hydroxy acids—which have been found to reduce the appearance of wrinkles—are also plentiful in peach juice.

The fiber structure of the peach contains plenty of pectin, along with the delicate cellulose network, and associated with it all are the fruit-cell contents that include the beta-carotenes and the polyphenolics. There are also some sugars—small amounts of glucose and fructose, larger amounts of sucrose, and probably some oligosaccharides.

As is true of all whole fruits, potassium is more abundant in peaches than sodium, which further adds to their value as a summer refreshment. The potassium from fruits, such as the peach, is needed to replace the potassium we lose in perspiration, especially during exercise. And the beneficial potassium-sodium ratio is also good for lowering blood pressure.

Perfectly ripened fresh peaches are available only in the heart of summer. Dried peaches are available all year long. Provided they have been prepared without any additives, dried peaches contain all the nutrients found in the fresh fruit, but in a more concentrated form. The vitamin-C content is diminished, but, because there are so many polyphenolics present, it is likely that vitamin C is there, bound to polyphenolics. Those polyphenolics also have amazing power to bind with sugars and their polymers, and to alter sweetness. As with dried apricots, dried peaches are surprisingly less sweet tasting than the fresh fruit and this is probably why.

Pears

Pears have an amazing power to refresh and heal. I learned this early on in Britain from one of our family stories. My father was only in his twenties when he was diagnosed with a duodenal ulcer and was lying in the hospital at death's door. Fortunately, a visitor brought him some ripe pear, carefully peeled and sliced. Somehow he found the strength to eat it and that began his recovery.

Pears are a delicately flavored fruit that nevertheless supply fruit benefits. The fiber content is unusual. In foods, lignin is present in very small amounts; it is, after all, a woody substance. But more is found in pears, especially in varieties that have a granular texture towards the center around the core—those granules are mostly lignin. Pectin is present in amounts comparable with apples and there is a quota of cellulose. There is a little glucose and sucrose in pears, but their sweetness mostly comes from fructose. The way in which pears brown after cutting reveals the presence of colorless polyphenolic antioxidants. The potassium content is high, but most other minerals and micronutrients, such as the B vitamins, carotenes, and vitamins C and E, are all present in small amounts. Of course, these small amounts become important when you eat several pears or eat them dried and in quantity. Evidently, it is just this combination of nutrients in the fresh pear that can be so reviving to someone who has become dehydrated during exercise or due to illness.

Plums and Prunes

Farmers' markets are wonderful places to learn about fruits and vegetables. At one near our home, I had my first taste of the French prune plums that are grown and converted to prunes here in California. Prunes are not just *any* kind of plum that has been dried. Fresh prune plums are incredibly sweet tasting and are chosen for drying because they have such a high sugar content. They have a yellow flesh and a dark golden purple skin. I say golden purple because there are flecks of shining gold to behold in the sun, on the blue-black surface of the prune plum.

Prune plums can be simply sun-dried, but I have also heard that the fresh fruit can be first dipped in a hot solution of diluted alkali, and then spread out to dry in heated sheds. The hot dip ruptures the skin to allow faster loss of moisture, but the disadvantage here is that some valuable polyphenolics could be leached out. In either case, the resulting well-dried plum is hard and unappealing. Prunes usually need to be remoistened to have an attractive texture, but still have a low enough moisture content to preserve them.

Sometimes sorbitol, naturally present in small amounts, is added to further improve the texture of plums. Sorbitol is closely related to glucose, but is not digested until it reaches the colonic bacteria. It acts as dietary fiber and contributes only half the calories of a digestible carbohydrate, such as glucose. The malic acid in plums also acts as dietary fiber and stimulates a healthful fermentation in the colon. The dark brown color of prunes suggests that the polyphenolics have been released from the cells during the drying process and have been oxidized, and combined with the cell fiber. The nutrients in the original plums are all concentrated in the prunes. They contribute B vitamins and minerals, especially potassium, and small amounts of beta-carotene. The laxative properties of prunes are due to the effects of the soluble fiber, the sorbitol, and the malic acid, and the favorable way they stimulate the colonic lactobacteria and bifidobacteria.

In plums, which generally contain fewer simple sugars than the prune plums, glucose and fructose predominate. Part of a plum's tartness is due to the rich supply of colored polyphenolics in the dark red skin. The fiber, vitamin, and mineral content of *all* plums is similar, and they all have a reputation for being laxative and helping with proper colon function. The high content of polyphenolics make plums a particularly valuable source of antioxidant protection.

Raspberries

The magnificent fragrance and flavor of raspberries makes them as attractive as they are health-giving. What a wonderful thing to discover that fruit, and raspberries especially, are so good for you that you never need to feel guilty about eating them. Few people grow their own raspberries, so the price might be high because they are so expensive to harvest. In the end, though, raspberries are well worth all you can spend on them.

Fresh raspberries eaten whole yield oils from the seeds as you crunch them, as well as fiber and cell juices. If the seeds are bothersome, they can be strained after the fruit has been softened by boiling in a small amount of water for thirty minutes or so. Boiling dissolves the oils and polyphenolics from the seeds, but does not diminish the polyphenolic content of the juices. In fact, the full raspberry flavor becomes richer because the final juice is more concentrated, and is slightly thickened by the most soluble fiber.

Because of the plentiful polyphenolics they contain, the antioxidant power of raspberries ranks very high, just below strawberries and above plums, and there is a generous amount of vitamin C, well conserved by these antioxidant polyphenolics. Raspberry seeds boost the B vitamins supplied by the fleshy part of the fruit, and raspberries are especially rich in folate, the anti-Alzheimer's vitamin.

Strawberries

Imagine being required to eat a pint of fresh strawberries every day for a month. The participants in one of our studies for the Strawberry Board found it an easy task and delighted in reciting how well they felt as a result. In turn, we watched to see whether all those polyphenolics and the folate in strawberries could be tracked in the blood. Sure enough, the folate levels rose and stayed higher. The polyphenolics were a little more difficult to assess because they enter the blood very rapidly and leave just as fast to spread out into the many different tissues of the body. They do, however, build up in concentration all through the body to provide anti-cancer protection and give antioxidant protection to nerves, skin, and the cardiovascular system. Large amounts of one particular polyphenol, ellagic acid, has been isolated from strawberries, and is especially potent in the prevention of cancers.

The extra-high folate content of strawberries is probably due to the little seeds on the outside of the fruit, and the vitamin-C content of strawberries is higher than oranges or kiwis. The fiber of the fleshy fruit is a mixture of cellulose, pectin, and other soluble fiber, and as a result, fresh whole strawberries make a wonderful purée.

Watermelon

Watermelon season coincides with the hottest days of summer. Perhaps watermelons are most refreshing to the very people who produce them, the farmers in the field in the heat of summer. The revival power of watermelon on a sizzling hot day is unsurpassed.

There is very little fiber in the flesh of the watermelon, but enough to hold more than 90 percent water. The minerals, potassium especially, and the sugars (3 percent sucrose, 2 percent fructose, and 1 percent glucose) present with the water help stave off the dehydrating effects of heat. In the presence of fiber, the sugars give a controlled, rather than sudden, boost to the glucose in the blood. In the heat stress of summer, it is important to take in plenty of antioxidants as an antidote, and watermelon makes a valuable contribution.

There may be many polyphenolic antioxidants present in watermelon, but the most valuable antioxidant discovered to date is the carotene lycopene. Also found in tomatoes, lycopene contributes to watermelons' deep red color. It is known that lycopene tends to accumulate in the lungs and prostate, giving anti-cancer protection to those tissues especially. There is a generous amount of carotenes in watermelon, also small amounts of the B vitamins, and some vitamin C.

Watermelon is usually served in large pieces for the purpose of quenching thirst, but perhaps its most useful nutrient is potassium. As is true of all the fruits and vegetables you eat, watermelon will give you a high potassium intake to balance with sodium, and a diet that is much richer in potassium than sodium is conducive to reduced blood pressure.

An Almost Endless List

The number of fruits that could be described here is almost endless. Some of them are particularly superb, and all deserve a place in our diet, but describing them all is beyond the scope of this book. Always remember that fresh fruit is a desirable food high in many protective compounds and energy from sugar that is balanced with fiber.

22

What's with Fiber in Vegetables?

From Flowers to Fruits, Leaves, Roots, and Stems

Ah, vegetables—the glory of the farmers' market! Chard, kale, spinach, bundles of herbs, and lettuce all neatly stacked and dutifully sprayed with water to keep them in freshly picked splendor. Broccoli, cabbage, carrots, garlic, onions, potatoes, and turnips piled in profusion. Artichokes, beans, beets, celery, cucumbers, fennel, okra, parsnips, squashes, and tomatoes in every corner of the display, every one qualifying as a vegetable, regardless of whether it is a flower, fruit, leaf, root, or stem.

With the notable exception of cucumbers, salad greens, or salad tomatoes, most vegetables are cooked before being eaten. Cooking uses the huge amount of water already in the fibrous plant cells to burst them open as it begins to boil and steam. Colored and flavored juices you would not otherwise taste are spread out in the softened fiber matrix. The cooking process makes the nutrients more available, besides making some vegetables soft and edible when they would otherwise be ignored. Very watery cooking methods, such as boiling greens, allow highly soluble nutrients, such as the B vitamins, to spread into the cooking water. If the water is then drained off, these nutrients are lost, so it would be better to eat them as part of a soup. Methods such as roasting, steaming, and stir-frying use the vegetables' own water and the nutrients remain in them. Ideally, people need to consume both raw and cooked vegetables, and possibly supplement the whole plants with vegetable juices, but not replace them.

Whole grains top the list for antioxidant power, with fruits next, and vegetables last. In defense of both fruits and vegetables, they contain so much more water than grains that, if the antioxidant power in the *dried* fruit or vegetable were measured, it would be comparable to, or better than that of whole grains. Vegetables are rich in beneficial phytochemicals and vitamins and each one has a different and useful contribution to make.

Bulb Vegetables

Onions and leeks qualify nicely as bulbs. The bases of their long leaves are swollen and layered into a bulb, with stored carbohydrate nutrients. A garlic bulb or clove, is also produced at the base of a leaf, but groups of leaves produce separate cloves which can each produce a new plant. All those stored carbohydrates in bulbs have been manufactured by photosynthesis in the upper green leafy structure and carried to the bulb ready for the growth of a new plant in the following year.

Fennel

The plant family that includes fennel (*Apiaceae or Umbelliferae*) also includes angelica, anise, caraway, carrots, celery, chervil, coriander, cumin (cilantro), dill, licorice, lovage, parsley, and parsnips. Fennel is a carminative, as are anise, caraway, coriander, and dill, which simply means it is a digestive that helps relieve gas, and induce burping. The New England Puritans chewed fennel during church services, presumably as a breath freshener.

A taste for fennel is worth acquiring, although the slightly licorice flavor of fennel is not always appreciated among Americans who remember childhood medicine flavored with licorice, anise, or fennel. Italians, on the other hand, who grew up eating fennel as a vegetable or salad, consider it wonderfully warming and delicious in flavor. The same is true for Eastern Europeans, who are accustomed to dark whole wheat and rye breads flavored with caraway, coriander, anise, or fennel seeds.

Fennel contains soluble and insoluble fiber, a good supply of B vitamins, some carotene, plenty of potassium, and flavor compounds that have been used since Roman times to soothe the digestive system and reduce gas.

As the seasons change, fennel is often eaten instead of celery and it can be prepared similarly. In a memorable cooking class a few years ago, author and chef Deborah Madison prepared a simple, superb dish of beets baked with fennel.

Garlic

Even in its mature form, garlic contains 64-percent water, which is enough to roast it whole, to deliciously tender morsels. The harsh, yet appetizing, flavor of raw garlic mellows to flavorsome sweetness when cooked and imparts its appetizing qualities to other, relatively bland, vegetables. A friend encourages her teenage children to eat kale by always dressing it with garlic and olive oil.

Garlic is perhaps the most potent health-promoting vegetable of all. The sulfur-containing compounds that contribute the most to garlic's flavor are physiologically active compounds and very strong antioxidants. When eaten frequently and in quantity, garlic has known anti-cancer and antibiotic benefits, and can help reduce cholesterol and protect against intestinal worms.

In light of the current fight against the diabetes that can follow obesity, it is interesting to note that the ancient Egyptians, Greeks, and Romans used garlic as a treatment for diabetes, and these treatments have all been verified in current studies. Eating a good deal of garlic can lead to a reduction of the fasting glucose level and an improvement in skin circulation. The only adverse effects of eating large amounts of garlic can be a thinning of the blood, so it takes longer than normal to clot, plus the odor of garlic on the breath. But if everyone around you is eating garlic, then this is not a problem. The blood-thinning quality also gives garlic a role in the prevention of strokes.

The sulfur compounds in garlic are embedded in fiber, and there is a high proportion of potassium and sufficient B vitamins to mobilize the large amount of starch (14.7 percent) present. The fiber in garlic includes a high proportion of soluble fiber (3.2 percent) compared with the insoluble (0.9 percent) fiber. Most of the soluble fiber is inulin, which is not digested but instead supports a healthy growth of bifidobacteria in the colon. The quantity of inulin taken in with large amounts of garlic eaten as a vegetable may be the most important reason for the cholesterol-reducing properties of garlic. The absorption of short-chain fatty acids from the colon as a result of inulin fermentation will result in favorable blood-cholesterol profiles. Extracts of garlic that do not include all of this inulin may not be as effective in reducing blood-cholesterol levels as garlic itself.

Onions and Leeks

The flavorful heart of most traditional dinners is garlic, onions, or leeks if you are eating a traditionally Welsh or Irish dinner—the leek is even the patriotic emblem of Wales. This is fortunate for our health, because garlic, leeks, and onions are major contributors of protective compounds.

In Holland in the early 1990s, onions were involved in one of the first definitive studies on antioxidant polyphenolics. Actual amounts of some major polyphenolics (quercetin especially) in the diet were measured and found to be large enough to have an effect. In the Dutch diet, these antioxidant polyphenolics were mostly obtained from black tea and onions (apples, too, but on a much lower level). Onions are especially protective against digestive tract cancers of the colon, stomach, and rectum.

The antioxidant polyphenolics are important for protection against stomach cancer, but are not the only factor protecting against other cancers. Inulin encourages good bifidobacteria to grow in the colon and increases acidity there. It is richly present in onions and is known to be protective against colon and rectal cancers. Additionally, the production of short-chain fatty acids from inulin in the colon is a likely explanation for the cholesterol-lowering properties of onions. As with garlic, onions have sulfur-containing compounds that make them beneficial for people with diabetes, particularly by reducing levels of fasting blood sugar.

The particularly protective effect of onions against prostate cancer has been validated recently. The incidence for breast cancer closely parallels that for prostate cancer. The French eat enough onions and garlic to have shown that breast cancer can be reduced by eating onions and garlic. Since first learning about this, a vegetable from the onion family has been an essential part of dinner in our house every single day.

Flower Vegetables

Flowers are generally thought of as decorative, or as passing in favor of the fruit that they will produce. All that beauty and reproductive power must surely contain some products useful to people, and indeed there are flowers that are eaten as vegetables. Usually the flowers are still in the bud and often not as recognizable as the wide-open flower would be. Artichokes, broccoli, and cauliflower are good examples of vegetable flower buds. There are also selected beautiful flowers, which are edible, such as calendula, the peppery nasturtium flower, or squash flowers. They can be wonderful additions to a salad or other dishes, but caution is advised because some flowers are *not* edible and, as with any other plant, they could be toxic. There are a number of good books on the subject, including *Edible Flowers* by Cathy Wilkinson Barash, which describes over fifty edible flowers, with great recipes.

Broccoli

Broccoli heads are essentially flower buds, and that's where the most biologically active compounds are concentrated. As with cabbage, broccoli has an important role in cancer prevention, heart protection, and stroke reduction.

In varieties of broccoli with thick stems, they can be put in to steam before the broccoli heads so they will cook longer. This stem material is a good source of soluble fiber and potassium, and if the whole stem is eaten, the fiber will include a high proportion of cellulose.

Broccoli heads are rich in carotenes for eye health. Antioxidant polyphenolics that protect against cardiovascular disease, anti-cancer compounds containing sulfur, and other anti-cancer compounds known as indoles are also found in broccoli, as well as cabbage. In the case of the healthful sulfur-containing compounds, these are made more available in the raw broccoli heads by a naturally occurring enzyme. Broccoli is one of the richest vegetable sources of vitamin K—it contains more than fresh cabbage.

Cauliflower

Although cauliflower lacks the green color and is low in carotenes, you can tell by its aroma that the anti-cancer sulfur-containing compounds are present, as are the antioxidant polyphenolics. The fiber is a good balance of soluble and insoluble, and, as in all the brassica vegetables, the soluble fiber, especially, supports favorable lactic bacteria in the colon. Cauliflower supplies noteworthy amounts of folic acid, potassium, and vitamin C.

Globe Artichokes

Dinner for my husband, Gene, is immediately festive when artichokes are on the menu. All you need to do to prepare them is to cut off the thorny ends of the leaves and rinse them. They are delicious raw, but even better when tenderized by steaming and eaten leaf by leaf until reaching the flower center, or choke (they are, after all, giant thistles just about to bloom). The leaves (sepals) on artichokes are a part of the flower, but since they are green and leaflike, that's what most people call them. The choke is edible only in very young artichokes. In older ones, it is far too coarse and needs to be cut out before eating the heart (the flower base).

Artichokes have an extraordinarily sweet aftertaste, following a somewhat bitter first impression. Polyphenolics abound in artichokes and seem to partially account for their flavor and their dual use as food and medicine, which has been recorded since Roman times, when extracts of artichoke were prescribed to increase the excretion of bile, as an antitoxin for the liver, as a diuretic to correct urinary problems, to prevent arteriosclerosis, and to treat itchy skin conditions. This measures up well with some of today's findings, such as the especially beneficial effect that artichokes have on the liver, and the reduction of LDL cholesterol. This could be due to the presence of a rare group of polyphenolics known as sylmarin, which was originally recognized in another thistle, milk thistle. Sylmarin is strongly anti-inflammatory, antioxidant, and anti-cancer, and has been successfully used to reverse liver damage.

Artichokes contribute to our daily needs, including the need to constantly replenish a variety of polyphenolics. Readily digested carbohydrates in the form of simple sugars are present in small amounts. Fiber carbohydrates are mostly soluble in the parts of the artichoke that are eaten, and include inulin fructooligosaccharides, which is the source of the surprisingly sweet aftertaste of artichokes.

The B vitamins are well represented, including folate, which is generously supplied—there are approximately 80 micrograms of folate per medium-sized artichoke. More than 400 micrograms of folate in the diet (an adequate amount) leads to beneficially low homocysteine in the blood, which, in turn, is associated with a low incidence of Alzheimer's disease, cardiovascular disease, and diabetes. The level of potassium is ten times higher than sodium so, provided you don't oversalt the artichoke, it can contribute to lowered blood pressure.

Fruit Vegetables

It's true that most fruits are sweet and are eaten as dessert, but some notable exceptions are cucumbers, okra, peppers, squashes, and tomatoes that are definitely fruit vegetables, having developed directly from a flower. The difference seems to be they are not particularly sweet, yet they provide color or texture to the first or second course of a meal, and are now recognized for their nutritional value.

Cucumbers

Ever since staying in a youth hostel in Norway in the 1960s, where breakfast consisted of cucumbers, dark bread, and buttermilk, I have eaten cucumbers for breakfast in a similar style, especially in the winter when good tomatoes are unavailable. I am also extremely partial to cucumber salad with dill and a dressing of oil, vinegar, honey, salt, and black pepper. But are cucumbers worth so much attention? My mother used to tell us that her physician in the 1920s said cucumbers were nothing but water. True enough. Cucumbers are extra high in water content (96 percent)—most vegetables contain about 88 percent. Concerning measured antioxidants, cucumbers are at the bottom of the list, below celery, lettuce, and potatoes. There *are* antioxidants and other valuable nutrients in cucumbers, but they are simply watered down—if the amount of water in each is taken into consideration, they can even match cabbage.

Cucumbers are good for fermenting into pickles, which indicates the presence of both fermentable sugars and fermentable soluble fiber, and the crispness of the pickled cucumber indicates that it has retained the unfermented cellulose fiber. Potassium is well-supplied in the fresh cucumber, but since salt is involved in pickling cucumbers, the increased sodium content erases the ability of the potassium in the fresh cucumbers to control blood pressure. The B vitamins, including folate, the carotenes, and vitamin C are all present in cucumbers.

If your local farmers' market includes a specialized cucumber farmer, as ours does, then you may find yourself eating and enjoying cucumber salad more often. Rest assured that even watery cucumbers have nutrients and they will contribute to your good health.

Okra

Okra must be mentioned because it is a fruit vegetable filled with the gummy soluble fiber that makes the Creole gumbos of the South so appetizingly thick and delicious. Okra does, in fact, contain more fiber than most vegetables, and the extra amount is mostly the mucilaginous soluble kind, plus some insoluble lignin. The other nutrients in okra consist of modest contributions of the B vitamins, carotenes, and vitamin C. Intriguing to me was that the mucilaginous fiber in okra contained glucosamine. Shellfish shells are the usual source of glucosamine, which is sold as a dietary supplement to relieve painful joints in osteoarthritis, but here is a vegetable food that contains this glucosamine naturally. Gummy okra juice has long been used in Asian medicine to sooth stomach irritation and inflammation. Recently, Swiss researchers verified its value. Fresh okra juice prevented the ulcer-causing bacteria, *Helicobacter pylori,* from settling on the stomach wall.

Olives

Table olives that seem to taste the best are prepared from ripe black olives that are bruised or split and soaked in a brine, in order for a lactic fermentation to occur. Ripe olives are unusual in that they contain significant amounts of mannitol, related to the sugar mannose, and this is readily fermented by the lactic bacteria (*Lactobacillus plantarum*) present in vegetable fermentations. It seems that all fermentations of vegetables are best done with the naturally occurring mixture of microorganisms, rather than with a single species, and for olives this often includes yeasts. In Egypt it is common practice to use a portion of old brine from a previous fermentation that is already rich in a naturally occurring mixture of lactic bacteria and yeasts.

The astringency of olives is attributed to oleuropein, which is a combined phenolic and sugar compound. But several other phenolics contribute to the astringency and color. Both the ripening and the acidic fermentation process mellow the flavors considerably. The alternative alkaline processing, for canned olives, removes or degrades a high proportion of the phenolic compounds. When processed in this way, the flavor of the olives becomes bland, and the health benefits are lost.

The flesh of the olive contains large amounts of oil, and after it is extracted, the remaining pomace is generally used only as animal feed or compost. The aqueous fraction extracted from the olive at the same time as the oil contains large amounts of water-soluble phenolic compounds. This is often discarded, but some enterprises concentrate these water-soluble polyphenolics for use as a medicinal antioxidant mixture. The oil fraction has a mellow flavor and still contains some of the oil-soluble polyphenolics, which preserve the oil against oxidation. The polyphenolics in olive oil give it healthy properties far beyond those for the oily components alone. Olive oil is in itself beneficial. It is more than 50 percent monounsaturated, and has fewer saturated (16 percent) and polyunsaturated (11 percent) components. A variety of vitamin-E tocopherols are also associated with the oily fraction from olives.

Peppers

Freshly roasted red chili peppers were hanging from every stand at the farmers' market we visited one September in Santa Fe, New Mexico. Some chili peppers were even being roasted right there in the marketplace, where they created a great feeling of hungry excitement as the pungent, fruity aroma wafted out.

Hot peppers are mostly added to foods in small amounts for their intensely hot flavor, which is due to a substance called capsaicin. Not surprisingly, this same substance can numb pain, especially on the skin, and hot-pepper extracts are part of many muscle-soothing lotions and creams.

The related sweet bell peppers are eaten in much larger amounts. Besides fiber, the most beneficial nutrients recognized in peppers to date are carotenes, which rival spinach in quantity, folate, potassium, and vitamin C.

Squashes

Buttercup, butternut, hubbard, kabocha (similar to butternut), and spaghetti squashes appear in the fall. They are truly astonishing in flavor and in their ability to have grown to such a size and quality from a single seed in just one season. The buttercup and kabocha are deliciously sweet and easily convert from a vegetable to dessert. Squash flowers are eaten as a delicacy, but they have an added bonus in that they contain a waxy sterol with anti-cancer potential.

By their inside color, which is bright orange or yellow, squashes are evidently rich in carotenes (3,360 micrograms per 100 grams). The retina of the eyes benefit from a rich supply of carotenes, particularly lutein and zeaxanthin, which are concentrated in the macula right at the center of the retina. Macular degeneration is much less likely to occur if the diet is rich in lutein and zeaxanthin, and butternut squash supplies substantial amounts of lutein and also some zeaxanthin. Although both kale and spinach have even higher amounts of lutein and zeaxanthin, no other orange or yellow fruits have as much of these two carotenes as butternut squash.

Squashes are sometimes regarded only as a vegetable for Thanksgiving, but they are rich in nutrients as well as flavor and can be enjoyed several times a week when in season. We find that the flavor and texture of buttercup squash, for example, is perfect just as it is, without any dressing, although various concoctions are delicious, such as the mixture with parmesan cheese and nutmeg used in the stuffed pasta *tortelli di zucca.* There is some starch (3 percent) in buttercup squash, but this is considerably less than in white potatoes (16 percent). The sweet flavor due to sugars (4.5 percent) is equally divided between glucose, fructose, and sucrose. There is 0.7 percent soluble fiber in the total of 1.6 percent fiber. The B vitamins and vitamins C and E are present in sufficient amounts to make a valuable contribution to our daily needs.

Melon, Pumpkin, and Squash Seeds. The seeds from various squashes, and the related pumpkins and melons, are extraordinarily nutritious. The South Americans were the first to eat pumpkin seeds, and now, in every country where squashes are eaten, the seeds are too. A friend introduced me to some gently roasted Chinese melon seeds. They had a slightly salty, anise-flavored coating that made them tempting to crack with my teeth to extract the delicious kernel. The kernels of pumpkin seeds contain the full range of nutrients expected from a seed kernel, including the B vitamins and vitamin E. They are also high in fiber, they contain starch and very little sugar, and their mineral content, especially magnesium, phosphorus, and potassium, is high.

Their 46-percent oil content makes pumpkin seeds extraordinarily oily. Pumpkin-seed oil is valued as a salad oil, especially in Austria and Hungary. Vitamin E is extracted along with the pumpkin-seed oil, which is high in polyunsaturated oils. During the extraction, an oil-soluble lignan is brought into the oil from the shell of the pumpkin seed. Lignans, also found in flaxseeds, are valuable anti-cancer agents, especially against prostate and breast cancers.

Tomatoes

The tomato, introduced by the Spanish into Naples in the 1500s, is certainly an essential part of Italian food. The Italians always held the tomato in high esteem, naming it *pomodoro,* the golden apple, but now it ranks as a staple throughout the entire Western world. Pizza, focaccia, pasta sauces, salads, and ketchup—a selection from these makes tomatoes a daily contributor to practically everyone's diet. Tomatoes are very healthy too, and well worth enjoying in quantity.

Lycopene was first found in tomatoes and its name is derived from the Latin for tomatoes, *Lycopersicon esculentum.* Although vitamin A can be toxic in too large amounts, the tomato provides controlled amounts of vitamin A from its precursor, beta-carotene, which is not toxic at all. Any excess beta-carotene or similar compounds in the tomato, such as lycopene, simply build up and get stored in the fat layers under the skin, which colors the skin varying shades of tan, and protects it from the damaging rays of the sun. The stored carotenes are released into the body as needed. Beta-carotene is also an antioxidant, as is lycopene, and these compounds are highly protective against cancers and cardiovascular disease, including those of the skin. The availability of the lycopene is enhanced by cooking the whole tomatoes. Lycopene is especially valuable in the prevention of breast and prostate cancers, and is best supplied by home-cooked tomatoes, commercially canned whole or pureed tomatoes, or tomato paste.

Nearly half the carbohydrates in tomatoes are dietary fiber, which makes them a low digestible-carbohydrate food. Tomato fiber, apart from the skin and seeds, is mostly soluble and, as anyone who has ever made tomato paste or sauce from a large quantity of tomatoes at the height of their season knows, there is a lot of water to evaporate off because tomatoes contain more than 90-percent water. The soluble fiber gives texture to tomato concentrates, such as pastes or sauces, and carries with it concentrated carotenes and lycopene.

Other vitamins that are concentrated with the soluble fiber in tomato sauce include folic acid and thiamine, as well as niacin, riboflavin, vitamin B_6, and vitamin E; the minerals, particularly potassium, also remain. The soluble fiber's value comes when it is finally broken down by the bacteria in the large intestine, producing short-chain fatty acids, such as acetic and propionic acids, that can be absorbed to regulate metabolism and cholesterol levels. A few calories will be derived from the soluble fiber as a result of this break-down by the bacteria, but very few will come from the insoluble fiber which basically passes through the body without being absorbed.

Leafy Vegetables

A healthful, delicious dinner should include a leafy green vegetable. Most people have grown up with this idea, but few have practiced it all their life. In our house, we have an evolving basic dinner design that currently begins with a leafy green salad for the first course, followed by a second course consisting of a whole grain, beans, a cooked leafy-green vegetable, an onion-family vegetable, an orange or red vegetable, and another vegetable in season, such as an artichoke or asparagus. Dessert is often homemade, Swedish-style cultured milk or yogurt and fruit or fruit concentrate, according to the season.

Until we became ardent shoppers at the local farmers' market, we were lax about eating greens other than salads containing lettuce and its relatives. Then we experimented with Russian, Italian, and curly kale, collard greens, chard, and beet greens. We had always eaten cabbage and spinach, but at the farmers' market other leafy greens were also there in tempting abundance, and we began to buy much larger amounts than we ever had in the supermarket. We learned that several of these greens could be grown year-round here in California by enterprising farmers, but the best season of all is the cooler spring season when these greens are at their sweetest and most tender.

There is a way, however, to make these greens appetizing when they are less than perfectly sweet and tender. After washing the greens, strip the leafy parts off the tougher stems. If the greens are tender before cooking, they'll be tender after cooking, too. If they are on the tough side, they can be finely chopped after cooking and served in a soup. To cook greens, simply stir them in a heated skillet or wok, with only a little water, until they wilt and turn bright green. They can then be dressed as a salad with olive oil, balsamic vinegar, salt, and pepper, and the addition of herbs or flaked dulse seaweed according to taste. Previously cooked onions, or garlic with ginger, can be added to give an entirely different, highly complementary effect. For traditional flavor ideas, we look into ethnic cookbooks.

Cabbage, Collard Greens, and Kale

Cabbage can be grown worldwide in any climate, but it is especially revered in Asia and Eastern European countries. Cabbage is in the *Brassicaceae* family, botanically classified with broccoli, Brussels sprouts, collards, and kale, and is often referred to as a brassica, or cruciferous, vegetable. The same botanical group used to be called the *Cruciferae,* or the mustard family. All have the characteristic four-petaled flower in common. Other edible plants in this family include arugula, canola (rapeseed), cauliflower, kohlrabi, mustard, mustard greens, radishes, rutabagas, turnips, and watercress.

The wrinkly Savoy cabbage, a highly developed vegetable dating at least from Roman times, was introduced into Roman Britain. But the Britains were already eating collards and the wilder dark-green kale, which they have continued to grow. They also grew the pale-green, smooth-leaved cabbage, which was developed in the colder climates of northern Europe and is the type preferred by the Germans, especially for making fermented sauerkraut.

The cabbage structure is dietary fiber, which is basically cellulose and pectin. There are antioxidant polyphenolics associated with the structural cell walls. Inside the cells, carotenes are in good supply (385 micrograms per 100 grams), as is folate (75 micrograms per 100 grams), but this cannot compare with the high quantities in kale or spinach (3,535 and 150 micrograms per 100 grams of carotene and folic acid respectively). The carotenes in kale are very rich in lutein and zeaxanthin, which are especially protective of the macular part of the retina in the eyes.

Cabbage has more vitamin C (49 milligrams per 100 grams) than spinach. Its value for preventing scurvy among Dutch sailors, who carried plenty of fermented cabbage on all their sea voyages, was recognized in the eighteenth century, long before vitamin C had been identified.

The characteristic cooking smell of cabbage is attributed to sulfur compounds, which also give the cabbage some of its most important health benefits. Studies show that people who eat cabbage and related vegetables are protected against bladder, esophageal, intestinal, and stomach cancers. This protection may be due to the sulfur-containing compounds, the antioxidant polyphenolics, or other concentrated compounds in cabbage, such as indoles. The leaf cells contain fatty substances, including essential oils, lecithin, sterols, and waxes.

Fermented cabbage can be stored through the winter, making it available even when the ground is covered with snow or is too frosty to cultivate. Initiation of the favorable lactic fermentation process in sauerkraut requires salt, usually 2.25 percent salt with respect to the weight of the cabbage. The salt is sprinkled on layers of cut-up cabbage and gradually dissolves in the water that is pressed out of the cabbage, under the pressure of a weighted lid. The required lactic bacteria are inherently present in small amounts on fresh cabbage, and take two weeks or more to multiply sufficiently to acidify the cabbage and make it into sauerkraut. Lactic and acetic acids are produced in large enough amounts to acidify and eventually, with the salt, preserve the sauerkraut from attack by unwanted bacteria. Sauerkraut is a source of favorable bacteria for the colon, and the fermentation increases the amount of vitamin K in the cabbage.

Sauerkraut has a reputation as a laxative and this is partially attributed to dextran, a glucose polymer produced from the fermented cabbage by *Leuconostoc* bacteria. Dextran is a soluble fiber that does not get digested, but remains viscous even when it reaches the bacteria of the colon. During fermentation, lecithin and the oils are broken down into their component parts. The oils give glycerol and fatty acids. Lecithin, a phospholipid important in building nerve tissue, gives glycerol, phosphate, fatty acids, choline, closely related acetyl choline, and lactyl choline, and these cholines are also believed to give sauerkraut some laxative properties. Choline is an essential part of nerve signaling, and is used to make lecithin and similar compounds throughout the body.

Lettuce

According to Beatrix Potter in *The Tale of the Flopsy Bunnies,* lettuce is soporific, to rabbits anyway. In my own experience, there is nothing so welcome to eat at the beginning of a meal than a lettuce salad, especially after being out backpacking for several days. Botanically, lettuce is in the *Asteraceae* family. Other closely related plants are artichoke, chicory, dandelion, endive, and radicchio. The medicinal milk thistle is also related. Apparently, original wild lettuce was appreciated for its milky sap, most evident when the main stem of lettuce is cut at harvest, and that is mildly soporific. In the early Roman period, lettuce was eaten at the end of the meal for its calming effect. This is quite different from our habit at home, where we seem to be appreciating the calming effect at the beginning of the meal. In France and Italy, and in some upscale restaurants, salad is served after the main course and before the cheese or dessert.

Lettuce is higher in vitamin K than either cabbage or spinach. Outside of that, however, the nutritional value of lettuce is disappointing compared to cabbage and spinach, but those lettuces with the deepest green leaves supply the most generous amounts of carotenes, folic acid, and potassium. The fiber content of lettuce is around 1.3 grams per 100 grams, which is relatively low, but is nevertheless a contribution to our daily needs. Lettuce is a gently flavored green leaf that is often eaten in quantity, and its special value may yet be found by looking again at the milky sap seen when it is first cut.

Spinach, Chard, and Beet Greens

Spinach (*Spinacia oleracea*) comes from ancient Persia and originally seems to have been much more widely used in the Middle East and eastern Mediterranean than cabbage. Spinach, long regarded as exceptionally healthful, has a super abundance of fiber, folic acid, and carotenes, especially lutein and zeaxanthin, and is also well-endowed with vitamin E and huge amounts of betaine. Although betaine has been known for a long time, it is now newly appreciated because, as with folate and choline, it has been found to reduce the homocysteine levels in the blood, leading to a reduced risk for Alzheimer's disease, cardiovascular disease, and diabetes.

The fiber in spinach, mostly cellulose and pectin-related substances, is much more abundant than in lettuce or endive. It is also rich in oligosaccharides, some of which are linked to antioxidant phenolics, which means that when they are finally digested by the bacteria in the colon, the phenolic compounds are released in the colon and will either be absorbed or will protect the colon. The oligosaccharides favor the multiplication of beneficial bacteria and this in itself is healthful, because short-chain fatty acids that can increase acidity in the colon are produced, and when absorbed, will lower cholesterol.

Beet greens and closely related chard are incredibly healthful, too. Beet greens are even better than spinach with respect to antioxidant power. In an Italian experiment, beet greens had an ORAC value of 2,442 units, whereas the value for spinach was 735. These were for fresh greens—after the beet greens and spinach were frozen, the values dropped to 308 for the beet greens and 420 for the spinach. The lesson here is to avoid frozen vegetables in general because they lose nutritional value as a result of processing. Only minimal cooking and preparation of the freshest leafy vegetables possible yields the maximum benefits.

Root and Tuber Vegetables

In the days of the pioneering immigrants, a digestible carbohydrate staple food supply that would last through the winter was essential. And it was the root and tuber vegetables, stored in the root cellar, that could be relied on as staples when grain harvests failed. Root and tuber vegetables are the food-storage parts of plants that can also be used to propagate new plants in the following season. They are nutritionally valuable even though they are not quite as bountiful in their supply of B vitamins as seeds, and they usually have very little vitamin-E tocopherols, although sweet potatoes are a valuable exception. A mixture of root and tuber vegetables as staples is advantageous because some root vegetables have unusually concentrated nutrients—for example, beets with their rich supply of betaine, and carrots and sweet potatoes with their carotenes.

Beets

Beets are especially revered in Eastern Europe, where they are served as borscht, a deeply crimson-colored vegetable soup. Borscht is the national soup in the Ukraine, and is well worthy of such great appreciation.

Besides deep crimson, beets come in white and golden, and their green leaves with red stems are relished as a cooking green, with flavor and nutrients similar to spinach and chard. The sugar beet from which sugar is extracted is white, as is the German mangold-wurzel that is fed to animals.

All beets are rich in pectin, and the white sugar beets are one of the commercial sources of pectin. Apple pomace provides the best pectin, but when supplies ran low in the 1940s, citrus peel and beets were investigated as other commercial sources. Not all pectin is alike, however, and apple pectin keeps its reputation of having the best gelling power.

As a vegetable, the red beet is a winner, especially if it is picked when the sugar (sucrose) content is optimal, and the beets are extra sweet. The color is due to a polyphenolic compound found almost exclusively in beets, which differs from other red polyphenolic pigments, and is very valuable nutritionally as an antioxidant. The measured antioxidant power of red beets (840 ORAC units) is in the same range as broccoli (890), and is better than red peppers (731) or oranges (750). In the few studies conducted to date, beets have proved their worth as cancer-fighters and their ability to bring down homocysteine levels in the blood. The usual explanation for this latter effect is a generous folate content, and beets have as much folate as leafy green vegetables. Beets are especially effective in lowering homocysteine levels in the blood for an additional reason: they also contain a large amount of betaine, closely related to choline, which is essential for the healthy formation of cell membranes, a healthy liver, and nerve-signal transmission. Choline and betaine also perform a function similar to folate in removing homocysteine from the blood.

In the fibrous cell walls of the beet, with which all these health-giving nutrients are associated, there is slightly more cellulose than pectin. Raffinose, which is built from one molecule each of glucose, fructose, and galactose, is also a dietary fiber found in beets. Raffinose is not digested but is completely degraded by the colonic bacteria and yields short-chain fatty acids that favorably acidify the colon and are absorbed with good effect on our blood-cholesterol profile. Mannitol is another unusual fiber found in beet.

Beets, especially golden beets, are valued for pickling, no doubt due to the rich content of soluble fiber, which is easily fermented by lactic bacteria.

Beets have a unique role in helping to find out whether you are eating enough of the right kind of fiber. The first test is to see whether you have a comfortable daily elimination. The second test is to notice actual food transit time, which ideally will be one to two days. Because beets are so distinctly crimson, the elimination of the undigested part of beets is easily recognizable. So, if you remember when you ate your beets, you will be able to estimate your transit time by looking at the color of your stool. This is not the precise method you would use in a clinical trial, but it is good enough to learn whether or not you have a healthy transit time.

Carrots

Cooked and puréed, carrots are often the vegetable to which children are first introduced. Carrots are also the ones they are most likely to grow in a garden, with some adult help. And they are the first to be triumphantly yanked from the ground, rapidly washed, and eaten raw with gusto, right there in the garden.

Carrots are an indispensable soup vegetable and are equally essential raw, in a plate of mixed sliced vegetables ready for a yogurt-herb dip at a buffet. They are naturally sweetened with a mix of sucrose, glucose, and somewhat less fructose. Like beets and most root vegetables, carrots have a good supply of pectin fiber, along with insoluble cellulose fiber, in the root cells. The pectin will ferment well when it reaches the bacteria of the colon, and the short-chain fatty acids produced will be absorbed, which partially explains the ability of carrots to lower cholesterol levels.

Orange, red, and yellow carotenes are named for the carrots that so richly contain them. No other vegetable, or fruit, seems to top the carrot for carotene content, which ranges from 4,000 to 11,000 micrograms per 100 grams of carrot. By comparison, green leafy vegetables are in the 3,000-microgram range of carotenes per 100 grams of food, cantaloupes are in the 1,000-microgram range, and apricots are in the 300-microgram range.

Beta-carotene is considered one of the most valuable carotenes because each molecule is converted into two vitamin A (retinol) molecules. The conversion takes place in the small intestines, and probably the liver, where vitamin A is stored. Other carotenes can also be converted to vitamin A, but less efficiently, and in some cases they are not converted at all.

Carotenes were first extracted and named in the 1820s, but it was not until 1920 that vitamin A was discovered, and 1957 before beta-carotene was shown to be a precursor of vitamin A. The importance of vitamin A is that it keeps the eyes healthy; its presence in the retina, at the back of the eye, allows you to see, even in very dim light. From this comes the alternative name for vitamin A, retinol. Lack of adequate amounts of either vitamin A or beta-carotene in the diet will cause a severe drying of the eyes (xerophthalmia) that leads to blindness. Blindness from lack of vitamin A usually occurs when the diet is very limited and contains neither whole milk nor carotene-rich fresh vegetables. Whole milk and butter contain carotenes extracted from the grasses and leaves that the cow eats. Carotenes and vitamin A need a fat to dissolve them, which explains their concentration in butter and the cream of milk, and is a reason why enough good fat in the diet is also necessary for their healthy absorption. Unfortunately, there are some countries where the diet is so poor in carotenes that blindness does occur. Babies and children are the most vulnerable.

The eyes are not alone in benefiting from carotenes; the skin, the reproductive system and all the tissues that surround the various organs need vitamin A supplied in the form of carotenes. In large amounts, vitamin A is actually toxic, so the best way to keep up the supply without this problem is by eating lots of carrots and leafy green vegetables. Cooked vegetables yield more carotenes for absorption than raw vegetables that are eaten as chunks.

A large dose of carotenes has the remarkable benefit of coloring the skin. Some people like the effect because they look as though they have a nicely matured suntan, without the redness. (When the skin is colored yellow from jaundice, the effect is not attractive and includes a yellowing of the whites of the eyes, which does not occur from an abundance of carotenes.)

Carotenes that collect in the tissues give great protection against cancer, and the beneficial effects in reproduction are well-documented. Still, it was fascinating to hear the story told by a baker friend. When they were first married, he and his wife were hoping for children right away. But when they didn't conceive as planned, they began drinking generous amounts of carrot juice daily and went on to have four healthy children in quick succession.

Carotenes, such as lycopene, that do not convert to retinol but have antioxidant effects are valuable in their own right as anti-cancer agents, in stroke prevention, and in lowering cholesterol levels. Whole carrots have many more health-giving benefits than beta-carotene alone.

While carotenes dissolve most readily in oils and fats and are antioxidant, the polyphenolics that are also antioxidant will dissolve easily in water. This is a wonderful natural phenomenon that gives protection to the two parts of our system that cannot easily mix. Carrots have their share of antioxidant polyphenolics associated with the fibrous cell walls that protect the carrot root. When we eat the carrot, we have the benefit of these polyphenolics, as well as the fiber, carotenes, and all the other components of living plant cells, such as the potassium and calcium also generously present.

Jerusalem Artichokes (Sunchokes)

Apart from the sweet aftertaste, Jerusalem artichokes bear no relation to the common globe artichoke. The Jerusalem artichoke is a sunflower root that was originally eaten by the Indians in Canada. Instead of starch, Jerusalem artichokes are particularly rich in a fructose polymer known as inulin. It is the soft jelly that escapes from the tuberous root after cooking, and, apart from the interesting, somewhat crunchy texture after briefly cooking, the Jerusalem artichoke is a rare source of inulin in good amounts.

As mentioned earlier, inulin is a dietary fiber that it is not digested until it reaches the bacteria of the colon. It particularly favors the colonic bifidobacteria, which convert it to acetic and lactic acids. Acetic acid very effectively increases the acidity of the stools, and in so doing reduces the risk of colon cancer. Also the enhanced bacterial growth it promotes increases stool volume and favorably speeds the stools through the colon. The estimated caloric contribution of inulin is 2 calories per gram, which is half the value for a gram of starch when it is normally digested. By eating the whole root, usually thinly peeled but also often left unpeeled, you also take in some B vitamins and minerals, especially potassium. There are antioxidant polyphenolics in Jerusalem artichokes, which make their contribution to our daily need for these protective compounds. The polyphenolics in Jerusalem artichokes are colorless until the cells are ruptured or cut, and the exposure to air turns the polyphenolics brown or pink.

Parsnips

Baked parsnips have a spicy-sweet flavor reminiscent of fennel and celery, and while growing up in Britain in the 1940s and '50s, they were a welcome and delicious part of our Sunday dinner, especially during the winter.

The family of plants that includes parsnips, also includes anise, carrots, celery, and fennel. Parsnips are close to carrots in the sense that the root is eaten in both, but here the similarity ends, because parsnips contain very little carotene. They were grown in Europe as a staple food until they were replaced by the potato. Indeed, the main attribute of parsnips is as a vegetable source of starch (6 percent), supplemented by some sugars (6 percent), mainly in the form of sucrose. The fiber (5 percent) present in the root cell walls is a nutritionally valuable mixture of soluble and insoluble fiber. Comparison with the potato that replaced parsnips is interesting. The potato contains starch (16 percent), sugars (1 percent) and fiber (3.5 percent), so weight for weight, the potato contributes more calories and less fiber to the diet than parsnips.

Potatoes (Solanum tuberosum)

In 1537, the Spanish introduced potato tubers into Europe from the region now known as Colombia. They were first considered a curiosity that was largely resisted, but when grain crops failed, they became a crop to rely on, and when their acceptance was complete, they developed as a crop to grow instead of grains. They are now the fourth most important food crop in the world, after wheat, rice, and corn (maize).

As an alternative crop to grains, potatoes were introduced throughout Europe, and from there to colonial countries, including North America. But the effectiveness of potato production gave rise to a dependence on it, in Ireland for example, so that grain crops could be used as money-making exports. One problem of relying on potatoes as a staple crop is that they do not store well, they sprout or are damaged by mold within a year of harvest. Also, potatoes are high in moisture and considerable quantities must be eaten to satisfy nutritional needs. By contrast, if properly cared for, grains can be stored for several years without damage, and their low-moisture content makes them a concentrated food. The Irish reliance on potatoes alone, as a staple crop, resulted in the infamous potato famine of 1845 through 1848, when the potato crops were ruined by mold before they could be harvested, and grains were largely unavailable because of the export program. The Irish are probably still the greatest potato eaters. For the most part, their potatoes are simply peeled, boiled, and eaten with milk or buttermilk and salt as a dressing, but they also eat Irish boxty bread, which is a version of their once-traditional oat flatbread, made now with potatoes and a little wheat flour.

In the rest of Europe, only the Italians and Germans were quick to follow up on the Spanish introduction of potatoes. It was not until the eighteenth century, when French agronomist Parmentier popularized the potato in France after winning a contest to find a bread substitute, that the rest of Europe began growing and eating the potato in earnest.

Potatoes are nutritionally valuable, and have proportions of protein, starch, and B vitamins comparable with whole grains, although the fiber content is much less than in whole grains, especially when they are peeled. A large baked potato eaten with its skin provides 2.9 grams of fiber (1.7 grams insoluble and 1.2 grams soluble), but without the skin, it contains only about 2 grams of fiber (0.6 insoluble and 1.3 grams soluble). Whole wheat, in the form of two slices of whole wheat bread, supplies about 3.9 grams of fiber (3.2 grams insoluble and 0.7 grams soluble).

Apart from the skin, the fiber in potatoes is distributed throughout the fleshy part. Although nearly half of the vitamin-C content is in the skin, there is a fair amount of it present, enough to prevent scurvy among the ship-bound Spanish explorers of the sixteenth century. And potatoes contain lipoic acid, an antioxidant capable of improving glucose metabolism and reducing the effects of type-2 diabetes. Also, there is enough potassium present to encourage control of high blood pressure. Parmentier's substitute for bread is amazingly healthful. One note of caution, however: When preparing potatoes, any green skin and eyes should be removed, because that is where the sharply flavored and toxic compound known as solanine concentrates.

Sweet Potatoes (Ipomoea batatas)

Although sweet potatoes and potatoes were both first cultivated in Peru, perhaps as early as 8,000 B.C., they are completely unrelated. They are also completely unrelated to yams (*Dioscorea species*). Sweet potatoes are in the same plant family as morning glory, and produce bell-like flowers on a large vine. A surprisingly widespread staple in the tropics, sweet potatoes are thought to have been established in the wild by birds carrying the seed, as well as through trade and colonization. In the United States, they are mostly grown in the South, having originally been planted there by Louisiana Indians.

Most sweet potatoes are so tasty that they are simply baked or boiled and eaten with the skin, which increases their fiber value. Sweet potatoes contain approximately the same amount of starch as potatoes, but have more sugar, mostly sucrose, than potatoes. As the orange or golden color suggests, there are plenty of carotenes (3,930 micrograms per 100 grams) in sweet potatoes. If eaten as a staple, they become a major contributor of carotenes, and give protection against diseases of the eyes and skin. The fiber content of sweet potatoes is 2.3 grams per 100 grams, perhaps 3 grams per 100 grams if the skin is included. Except for the skin, the fiber is evenly spread throughout, in approximately equal amounts of insoluble and soluble fiber.

Valuable amounts of vitamin E are also present in sweet potatoes, giving them an even greater nutritional advantage over potatoes. Potatoes have more vitamin B_6, but even so, the B vitamins are well represented in the sweet potato, and it has just as much potassium as the potato.

Considering how tasty sweet potatoes are, it is surprising how seldom they are eaten. Perhaps the main reason is that they do not keep as well as potatoes. I have read they should not be refrigerated or they will lose their flavor, and they should not be kept in a warm place either, or they will sprout and ferment. Cellar-range temperatures, with plenty of ventilation, are about right. In the tropics, they probably dig them up and cook them right away.

Turnips

In the 1590s, after the grain famine in the city of London, turnips, carrots, and parsnips became very important, especially among the poor. The market gardeners seized the opportunity to provide root vegetables to Londoners, and from that time on, the diet, especially of the poor, included far more vegetables.

Turnips are a valuable source of dietary fiber, especially soluble fiber, but they contain only a little starch (0.2 percent), some sugars (4.5 percent), and a little vitamin C, which grains do not, unless they are sprouted. Turnips, in the venerable brassica family of vegetables, contain antioxidant polyphenolics and some of the highly protective sulfur-containing compounds that have given other brassicas, such as broccoli and cabbage, a good reputation for cancer prevention.

When turnips are used as a staple, instead of wheat, however, their limitations are revealed. In 1629, a London pharmacist noticed hunger edema (waterlogged tissues and swollen limbs) among the poor as a result of eating turnips as a staple. A lot of turnips must be eaten to provide enough digestible carbohydrate for people's energy needs because they are so high in water content (91 percent). Wheat and most grains supply a much more generous amount of starch and vitamin E than turnips and, provided they are eaten in the whole form, are much more healthful as a staple than turnips.

Compared with other greens, turnip greens are reputed to have a very high vitamin-K content (650 micrograms per 100 grams). Vitamin K is essential for blood coagulation.

Stem Vegetables

The stems of some vegetable plants have been selected by gardeners and farmers, and gradually improved over the centuries because they are so flavorful. Celery and asparagus come to mind first as stem vegetables, but exotic cardouns, which are stems from a type of artichoke, and rhubarb, which is usually eaten as a dessert, are also edible plant stems.

Asparagus

As an ancient Persian vegetable, asparagus, with its elegant spears, looks the part. The sight of asparagus on any plate is inspiring, and there is always a hint of luxury in the eating. Asparagus tips grow into fronds of asparagus fern, enjoyed in professional flower arrangements, but no longer desirable as food. Asparagus spears are used as a vegetable only while they are young and tender.

Because asparagus is mildly diuretic, due to the compounds that give it a characteristic flavor, it has often been considered a medicinal food. It has a high concentration of folic acid (175 micrograms per 100 grams), similar to the amount in leafy green vegetables, and small but significant amounts of the other B vitamins, plus carotene.

The sweetness of asparagus is partly due to the minimal amount of simple sugars present. There is also inulin, the sweet-flavored fiber known as a fructooligosaccharide, which favors the growth of the especially beneficial bifidobacteria. Asparagus contains both soluble and insoluble fiber, in equal amounts. There is also a good enough supply of polyphenolic antioxidants to give it an antioxidant rating comparable with raspberries.

Celery

Although most dietary fiber is anything but stringy in appearance, celery is probably the first vegetable to come to mind when dietary fiber is discussed because celery stems have cellulose strings. Cellulose plays an important role in forming the walls of the celery plant cells and maintaining their rigidity by holding large amounts of water (celery is 95-percent water). Mannitol is associated with the fiber in the cells of celery. This sweet-flavored soluble fiber is not digested until it reaches the bacteria of the colon, where it favors the growth of beneficial bacteria and produces short-chain fatty acids, which get absorbed and help give a favorable blood-cholesterol profile. Mannitol is also diuretic, which partially explains celery's reputation as medicinal. There are a few antioxidant polyphenolics, although barely more than in lettuce and cucumber. Celery has a generous amount of potassium that contributes to its reputation for lowering blood pressure. Research continues to determine which particular compounds in celery and celery seed account for its healing properties.

23

What's with Fiber in Seaweeds and Fungi?

Seaweeds

As a child, it was a pleasant revelation when I discovered it was okay to eat seaweed. It always seemed to be so enticingly edible when freshly washed in by the tide on the rocks of the northeast coast of England in the late 1940s, but nobody I knew seemed to be eating it.

Many years later, a Japanese neighbor proudly presented me with a sandwich of rice wrapped in nori seaweed, with a sour plum in the center, that was amazingly delicious. And in a Hawaiian-Japanese restaurant, we savored seaweed salad with at least three kinds of seaweed.

By that time, we had already developed our own preference for dulse, which is sold in neat packets from Maine. The flavor is reminiscent of salty anchovies, and the color is a gorgeous dark pink-purple. Dulse flakes sprinkled on kale or salad greens, along with an olive oil and balsamic vinegar dressing, add instant excitement. Tossed into soup, dulse leaves soften and add their slight saltiness and zesty seafood flavor.

The British have lost too much of their food culture, including a taste for seaweed, to industrialized food production. For millennia, seaweeds were part of the diet in British coastal regions, and the custom continued longest in Ireland and Scotland. In late nineteenth-century Ireland, dulse was relished with potatoes, and seaweed was prepared as a savory spread for toast and sold in London as a delicacy.

Seaweeds make a valuable contribution to the diet, beyond their flavor and texture. Apart from water, they are almost entirely dietary fiber, and practically all the fiber is soluble. This means the fiber is not digested until it reaches the bacteria of the colon. The short-chain fatty acids produced by bacterial fermentation can be absorbed and will contribute to a highly favorable blood cholesterol profile. The calorie contribution will be half that of a corresponding weight of starchy food.

Because it grows in the sea, the sodium in seaweed is usually much higher than the potassium, exactly the opposite of land plant foods, which have a higher amount of potassium, so seaweed is *not* helpful for lowering blood pressure. Even so, dried nori seaweed has exceptionally high potassium, which suggests that thorough washing can reduce the sodium content of seaweeds. Minerals, such as copper, iodine, iron, phosphorus, and zinc, are also present in larger amounts than in most land plants. When seaweed is eaten regularly, the valuable mineral iodine is contributed to the diet in sufficient amounts to prevent an enlarged thyroid gland, or goiter.

Two other impressive nutrients in seaweed are glucosamine and vitamin B_{12}. The vitamin B_{12} found in eggs, meat, and dairy is well-absorbed and these sources are considered ideal for it. Seaweeds also contain vitamin B_{12}, but according to some researchers, it comes in several forms and its usefulness cannot be relied on. For example, raw nori is a far more effective source of biologically useful B_{12} than processed dried nori.

Ever since learning that glucosamine is a valuable nutritional supplement for rebuilding joints damaged by arthritis, I have wondered where in the diet we would naturally obtain glucosamine. Even meat eaters do not eat much collagen, which is a source of glucosamine. Lactic bacteria in cultured milks, such as yogurt, sourdough breads, and fermented vegetables, such as sauerkraut, can be a significant source, if they are a major part of the diet. Seaweeds and mushrooms can contribute an important amount of glucosamine, and okra is valuable, too, especially if gumbo is eaten frequently. Baker's yeast cell walls contain only small amounts of glucosamine, so their contribution appears to be minor.

My grandmother in Britain had very painful arthritis, and I have often wondered why she, and thousands like her, should have had the disease at all. Was her diet to blame? My grandmother's diet, which was far from a whole plant-food diet, contained white bread leavened only with baker's yeast, and she did not seem to eat any fermented foods or seaweed. She was frugal with fruits and vegetables. Otherwise she ate meat and fish, used fresh milk, and often made cakes with white flour, white sugar, butter, eggs, and sometimes blanched almonds. Could it be that she never in her life ate foods that contributed enough glucosamine, especially when vitamin C and the polyphenolic antioxidants were also so low in her diet? Glucosamine is considered nonessential because the body can make it, but perhaps not always enough, so people should routinely be eating lactic fermented foods and seaweed or mushrooms that naturally contain glucosamine.

Fungi

People have said that mushrooms appear to be exotic and tasty, but they are not really necessary. Such a drastic statement begs rethinking, of course, and since I began searching for foods that naturally contain glucosamine, I have found that mushrooms are one of the very few foods that are actually rich in glucosamine. The advantage mushrooms have over seaweeds as a source of glucosamine is that they contain very little sodium and plenty of potassium, while the reverse is true in most seaweed. So, if you are concerned about improving your blood pressure, while increasing your intake of glucosamine, mushrooms prepared with little or no salt will be preferable to seaweed. A substantial portion of the total protein is incorporated into the structural fiber of mushrooms as either glucosamine or closely related materials. There are B vitamins present in mushrooms, including higher amounts of biotin, folic acid, niacin, pantothenic acid, and riboflavin.

Current studies are focusing on the possibility that mushrooms can boost immunity and have anti-cancer properties. So far, the compound lentinan, isolated from shiitake mushrooms, has shown some activity against colon cancer, and common mushrooms may turn out to contribute to the prevention of breast cancer, and stomach cancer as well.

Suddenly mushrooms seem highly desirable and worthy. There are a variety of mushrooms available to buy in addition to the common cultivated mushroom—oyster mushrooms, portobellos, and shiitake mushrooms, to name just a few. If you are fortunate enough to be near a local farmers' market that has a mushroom vendor, you will be able to try wild mushrooms, such as boletes or chanterelles, picked by experts when in season.

24

What about Extracts, Juices, and Teas?

Beyond Fiber—Plant Food Extracts, Juices, and Teas

There is a limit to the amount of fiber people can take. Over the millennia, the human digestive system has developed so it can handle only 25–50 grams of fiber per day, according to a person's height. Temporarily set aside the realization that many people eat too little fiber for reasons previously discussed: that refined wheat is practically fiber-free, and that people eat too few fruits and vegetables. Look instead into plant foods other than white flour that have been extracted from the whole plant source, olive oil for example, and see how they fit into the diet. Provided that most plant foods are eaten in the whole form as part of a plant-based diet, it is easy to take in the optimal amount of fiber. Beyond this, there are plants with tantalizing content, which people do not normally eat in the whole-plant form—maple trees, raw olives, sugar cane, tea leaves, and whole pomegranates, for example. In each case, the fiber is either too coarse for the digestive system, or the taste is too strong. Similarly, citrus peel, gum trees, and gum beans, provide edible soluble fiber, but no one wants to eat raw citrus peel in quantity, or a woody tree, or a hard gum bean. When foods are extracted from their original fibrous structure, many possibilities for variety in their preparation come to the fore.

Olive Oil

Black juicy olives look wonderfully appetizing and can be excellent eating if they are picked from the tree in June. More often, the olives are picked when they have just turned black, in the late fall or early winter, and these olives are intensely bitter. This is due to phenolics characteristic of the olives, which are powerfully antioxidant, and mostly water soluble. If the juice of the olive is squeezed out until only the fibrous skin and pit is left, and is allowed to settle, there will be a golden oily layer and a purple watery layer. It is this purple layer that contains most of the antioxidant phenolics. Other phenolics are soluble in the olive oil and protect it against rancidity, as well as provide protection against degenerative diseases. When olive oil is first separated after pressing, it is usually cloudy due to very fine droplets of watery olive juice suspended in the oil, but after six months, the oil clears and a purple deposit can be seen at the bottom of the bottle.

The olive oil separated from the fiber and most of the phenolics is a valuable source of oil. The Romans preferred it over any animal fat, and it is widely used in the Mediterranean countries. Judging from the health and longevity of the people in Crete, their diet is one of the healthiest of all the Mediterranean diets, and two staples in their diet are whole grains (barley and whole-wheat breads) and olive oil.

Normal considerations with oils are the proportions of monounsaturated, polyunsaturated, and saturated fats. Olive oil is mostly monounsaturated, but it contains both omega-6 and omega-3 polyunsaturated fats, and is extracted from a fruit, technically, rather than a seed, although in many pressing methods, the olive pit is also crushed and extracted for oil. Olive oil contains vitamin-E tocopherols, and has an especially high concentration of sterols that help make it protective against cardiovascular disease.

Other Important Oil Extracts

Many valuable oils are extracted from nuts and seeds: almonds, walnuts and other nuts, flax, safflower, sunflower, the seed of the pumpkin, even the seed of the tea plant. Oils are also extracted from the pulp of avocados and the fruit of the oil palm. All these oils are best unrefined, and when used in moderation and to replace saturated animal fats, are healthful additions to the diet.

Cane Sugar Extracts

The giant tropical grass known as sugar cane (*Saccharum officinarum*), has supplied people with a sweet juice and crystals of sugar (sucrose) since antiquity. One of the most ancient preparations from sugar cane, *gur,* is still made in India. A similarly produced unrefined whole cane sugar is known as *rapadura* in Brazil, *jaggery* in Nigeria, and *panela* in Columbia. Basically, the fibrous cane is crushed, and the extracted juice is clarified by filtration, then heated to evaporate much of the water, until crystallization of the sugar begins. Next, the thickened liquid is spread out on large trays to evaporate to a dry enough state to be ground for baking and table use.

To the consumer, the distinguishing characteristic of unrefined whole cane sugar is its brown color and the fact that it is coarse powder rather than crystalline. Crushing the cane to release the juice, the clarification step, and other details may be primitive or up to date, but unrefined whole cane sugar contains the maximum amount of nutrients from the sugar cane. The brown color and rich flavor of unrefined whole-cane sugar is indicative of antioxidant polyphenolics and, as with all plants, whole sugar-cane extract is rich in potassium. Jaggery, the Nigerian unrefined whole cane sugar, contains 285 milligrams potassium, 117 milligrams of magnesium, and 92 milligrams of calcium per 100 grams. Perhaps not surprisingly from a whole-plant extract, jaggery contains 8-percent starch with the 89-percent sugar, and although sucrose predominates, it also contains small amounts of glucose and fructose.

Molasses, the clarified concentrate of sugar-cane juice, still contains some of the sugar originally present, and most of the minerals and polyphenolics. For the production of refined cane sugar, the cane juice is concentrated until the sugar begins to crystallize, and at that point the brown liquid is centrifuged off. Colorless crystals are obtained by repeated solution in water and re-crystallization. Unless they have been crushed to a fine powder for use as confectioner's sugar, refined sugars can be recognized by their crystallinity. Adding molasses to refined sugar crystals to produce brown sugar is a common practice.

Fruit and Vegetable Juices

Ideally, whole fruits or vegetables are eaten without any of their parts being discarded, except perhaps some tough peel, tough stems, or hard seeds. However, when juices are extracted from fruits and vegetables, they are no longer a source of fiber in the diet. It is important to understand that, in the form of juices, fruits and vegetables become only supplements to the diet. They can be valuable supplements, but they are not whole-plant foods.

As supplements, these juices have tremendous value for their concentrated phytonutrients. After vigorous exercise, it is important to quench thirst, but it is also important to replace minerals that may be lost, as well as antioxidant plant polyphenolics, carotenes, and vitamin C, all of which are well supplied by fruit and vegetable juices. If you are concerned about increasing your ability to fight cancer, cardiovascular disease, and diabetes, then individual fruit and vegetable juices can provide concentrated amounts of disease-fighting nutrients, especially antioxidant polyphenolics and carotenes.

Fruit juices that are particularly rich in phytonutrients include blackberry, blueberry, cherry, cranberry, and raspberry juices. Vegetable juices rich in phytonutrients include those made with beets, carrots, celery, or tomatoes.

Fruit and vegetable juices are especially appreciated before and after vigorous activity, during pregnancy and lactation, when children are growing fast, and during illness.

Pomegranate (Punica granatum) Juice

The pomegranate is a gloriously decorative fruit, with a tiny golden crown, King Solomon's Crown, on top of a crimson orb. But it is very difficult to eat because the juicy seeds are buried in a bitter pulp and the skin is tough as leather. Eastern Europeans and the people of the Middle East treat the pomegranate as more than just decorative. There the seeds are separated from the pulp and used in salads and juice—the pomegranate is especially good for juice. A concentrate of pomegranate juice keeps well and is used as a part of a salad dressing (especially with walnuts), on rice, or diluted as a refreshing drink.

The pomegranate (*Punicaceae*) appears to be in a class of its own botanically and in its potential for healing. The crimson color indicates that pomegranate juice is very rich in antioxidant polyphenolic compounds—its measured antioxidant power is even higher than blueberries. Because of this high antioxidant power, pomegranate juice is beneficial in the prevention of cancer, cardiovascular disease, and diabetes. Although some vitamin C is present, along with small amounts of B vitamins, and potassium, the real value of the pomegranate is in the other phytonutrients it contains. When the juice is made, it can contain oils and extracts from the seeds and skins, as well as from the juicy pulp surrounding the seeds. The seed oils included in pomegranate extracts have great potential to reduce breast cancer tumors, and the phytoestrogen compounds found in the juice and seed oil give pomegranate juice the potential power to reduce the symptoms of menopause and its effects, including osteoporosis.

Teas

Aromatic green leaves of mint, flowers of hibiscus and chamomile, ginger root, licorice root, orange and lemon peel, or rose hips can all be steeped in very hot water to produce aromatic, flavorful herb teas. Each herb tea contains phytonutrients that invariably include antioxidant polyphenolics, and are often much more than simple refreshment or comfort. You can drink them when you have a cold or an upset stomach, if you can't sleep, or most of all when you're tired and still want to feel bright. Echinacea is good for a cold, as is ginger, which is also beneficial for an upset stomach, and chamomile helps bring on sleep. But most desired of all is the tea that keeps us awake and bright because it contains caffeine, the tea made from *Camellia sinensis,* known simply as *tea.* Tea is indigenous to Southeast Asia, and the leaves are prepared in a variety of ways. Whether a tea will be green or black is determined by how much the fresh moist leaf is allowed to ferment before drying, and how much oxidation takes place—when the polyphenolics released from the cells are oxidized, they turn black.

Green teas are the least fermented and oxidized, and their color is due to the large amount of polyphenolics that have not been oxidized. The result is that green teas provide more protective polyphenolics and less caffeine than black teas. Even though there is more available caffeine in black tea, and many of the polyphenolics are oxidized, it still contains a useful supply of protective polyphenolics. All tea leaves, green and black, are extraordinarily high in vitamin K, and the mineral potassium, and they, along with the caffeine and many of the polyphenolics, are all easily infused in hot water to make classic tea.

> Although we have mentioned only a few common extracts, juices, and teas, many more exist. Juices of fruits and vegetables, and teas are a valuable addition to a high-fiber, plant-based diet.

Soluble Fiber Extracted from Plants—Gums, Inulin, Pectin

Soluble-fiber gums are well known for giving a pleasant texture to prepared foods, such as ice cream, icings, milk shakes, pie fillings, processed cheese, salad dressings, sauces, and sherbets. These gums also stabilize foods for a longer shelf life, by preventing separation of the watery part of the formula. Pectin is best known for its use in making jam set well. Medicinally, isolated soluble fibers are useful as dietary supplements.

Gums

Guar gum, the soluble fiber located in the cotyledons (the two halves of all bean seeds) of the guar bean, is obtained directly from a bean long grown in India and Pakistan. In this era of cholesterol monitoring, there is a theory that the viscosity of the gum plays a part in binding cholesterol from food, so guar gum is often prescribed to lower cholesterol levels. Although cholesterol in the blood is reduced in a number of cases, this theory for its action is not well supported. Nor is the suggestion that cholesterol-related bile acids are bound by the gum and carried out of the digestive system. Guar gum remains undigested until it reaches the highly beneficial bifidobacteria in the colon (favored by guar gum), at which point it is completely digested, so the carrying and binding powers of the gum end soon after it enters the colon. Instead, the effectiveness of guar gum is usually attributed to the short-chain fatty acids, which are produced during complete fermentation in the colon. These short-chain fatty acids are readily absorbed from the colon, and they then exert a favorable influence on your metabolism, especially your cholesterol profile.

Sometimes guar and other gums are added to the diet in a mixture with insoluble fiber to increase stool volume and ease elimination. But the stool-bulking aspect of gums is minimal, their usefulness is due instead to the increased bacterial fermentation in the colon.

In addition to cholesterol lowering, guar gum has another medicinal function. It will reduce average blood sugar (glucose) in many cases, by slowing down the speed at which glucose can be absorbed. In this case, the most viscous guar gum preparations produce the greatest effects.

All the soluble-fiber gum preparations that are used medicinally will usually reduce both cholesterol and average blood glucose. For some people with diabetes, this means that the amount of insulin required can be reduced simply by taking a gum medicinally. Besides guar gum, there are other seed gums, from locust (carob) beans and psyllium seeds, that are used either medicinally or in food preparation. And the tree gums acacia and tragacanth, obtained from the tree or shrub bark, have medicinal properties similar to the seed gums. Xanthan gum is obtained from bacteria that naturally produce the gum, and it has similar medicinal properties.

The pleasant gumminess of oatmeal is due to beta-glucan, an indigestible carbohydrate (soluble fiber). Rye fiber contains beta-glucan and another gummy soluble fiber, pentosan, which accounts for the amazingly gummy texture of rye doughs. These fibers are sometimes extracted and used to texturize food or as a dietary supplement.

Seaweed, eaten as sushi, soup, or salad, offers a jellylike texture due to the nature of the fiber it contains, which is not digested until it reaches the bacteria of the colon. The gelling fibers, agar and carageenan, are extracted from seaweeds. (Agar is an exception here—it is an insoluble fiber-gelling material.)

Many beans and seeds, such as flax, contain carbohydrate gums that provide interesting eating texture, but very few calories because they lack digestibility. As a prime ingredient in Creole gumbo, okra gives an appetizing gumminess and stringiness to this soup. Okra gum contains protein as well as carbohydrate in its structure. It also includes glucosamine, which is not digested and behaves like dietary fiber, exciting news to anyone who uses glucosamine-type compounds to treat their arthritis or improve their cholesterol profile, and would like to obtain it from a plant source. Other plant sources for extracted glucosamine (as opposed to more usual shellfish sources) are certain fungi and green algae, such as chlorella. Although rarely mentioned, there's evidently much to learn about the presence of glucosamine and related polymers in these lower plants. The fungus used to make tempeh, the bacteria used to make natto from soybeans, and the baking yeasts, including those found in sourdoughs, all produce glucosamine-related fiber. Several of the bacteria found naturally in sourdough starters also produce fiber gums, even cellulose, as does the tea fungus, which is actually a colony of bacteria and yeasts.

Inulin

Chicory root is not usually eaten as a whole-plant food, but inulin-containing extracts from it have long been used in beverages. These extracts give mild flavor, slight sweetness, and a pleasing fullness of texture when added, for example, to coffee. Inulin is a fructooligosaccharide (FOS), which is a polymeric carbohydrate built from fructose that has gained recognition from consumers because it is added to commercial fermented milk products. Because the FOS encourages the growth of bifidobacteria in cultured milk products, it is seen as a very healthful addition to the diet. Jerusalem artichokes also contain inulin (FOS), which gives the artichokes a wonderfully sweet flavor and produces a soft, clear gel after cooking. The inulin polymer is particularly valuable because it promotes the production of bifidobacteria in the colon.

All the medicinal properties expected from a soluble fiber are seen for inulin. It acts as a laxative, and helps to lower cholesterol and reduce average blood sugar levels.

Pectin

Pectin, extracted from apples, forms a jelly with sugar and water. Pectin and cellulose are the common materials of plant cell walls, including apples, but there are hundreds of similar materials inside plant cells. The various combinations give us the gummy, jelly, or crisp textures of plant foods.

Pectin is good for making jams and jellies because, without it, the fruit would have to be concentrated further to produce a favorable firmness on cooling. Preferably, commercial pectin is isolated from apples, but more usually it is produced from citrus peel and sugar beets.

Pectin is a soluble fiber, but its structure differs from gums, which are polymers of sugar. To be defined as pectin, some of the sugars in the polymer have been naturally modified so they have an acidic character (uronic acids). Pectins differ from gums because of this acidity, which seems to aid in the absorption of such minerals as iron and zinc.

Pectins are used medicinally as an antidote to diarrhea because they promote favorable lactic bacterial proliferation in the colon. Short-chain fatty acids absorbed from the colon into the blood—the result of lactic bacteria fermentation of pectin in the colon—explains the reduction in LDL cholesterol. Pectin, like gums, reduces the average blood-sugar level.

When you take a look at all the diseases and problems, a powerful overall picture emerges, graphically outlining the key role that a plant-based diet high in fiber has in preventing them. And some of the weaker correlations between optimal health and a whole-plant food would no doubt disappear if the entire diet were looked at as a unit.

Epilogue

The key to building good health is to always eat grains in the whole form, beans, lentils, peas, and other legumes, nuts, oils with both omega-3 and omega-6 fatty acids, and plenty of fruits and vegetables, including leafy greens.

By constantly educating yourself to eat only the food that pleases *all* your senses and truly enhances your well-being, it becomes unimaginable that you would ever make the mistake of eating refined grains, refined sugars, or hydrogenated vegetable oils.

Appendices

Appendix A

Graphs of Carbohydrates, Water, Proteins, and Fats in Plant Foods

The completely digestible parts of plant foods are the starches, sugars, proteins, and fats, with fiber and water making up the rest, to approximately 100 percent. Vitamins, minerals, and polyphenolic antioxidants are tremendously potent in their action, but they contribute little to the overall composition of plant food. Also, since they are often embedded in the most fibrous parts, such as the skins and the embryonic plant, their amounts are proportional to the amount of fiber present. This is valuable information when you use the following charts to compare foods. Proportionately, the fiber may seem small compared with the starch, sugar, protein, or fat content, but the fiber effect is magnified because it is the carrier of so many vitamins, minerals, antioxidant polyphenolics and other phytonutrients.

For the record, carbohydrates are the *sum* of sugars, starches, and soluble and insoluble fibers (fiber is usually sugar polymer). Soluble fiber is not digested at all, but is attacked by the bacteria in the colon to yield some absorbable acids. And insoluble fiber is neither digested, nor attacked appreciably by the colonic bacteria. Therefore, using the formerly fashionable buzz words *low-carb* for a diet was meaningless. It would have been better to say *low-digestible-carb* diet, but that's too much of a mouthful so it was abbreviated to low-carb. A bar chart of refined wheat flour is included to compare with 100-percent whole-wheat flour. The whole-wheat flour is regarded as a low (digestible) carb option to refined wheat flour. With respect to the main nutrients, the differences in composition between the two are not dramatic. Instead, the really significant differences are the benefits to be derived from the nutrients carried along with the fiber found only in the whole-wheat flour—the vitamins, minerals, and polyphenolic antioxidants, many of which favorably limit the way that starches and sugars are used in the body.

All the whole-plant foods are usually allowed in various healthy weight-loss plans, because the whole food prevents the excessive rise and fall of blood sugar levels seen with refined sugar and refined flour foods. The polyphenolics in the whole plant are probably the most active in moderating the glycemic response. As mentioned earlier, in our studies we have seen this effect with raisins versus refined glucose. Raisins, rich in polyphenolics, give a sustained rise in blood sugar, whereas the same amount of plain glucose gives a rapid rise and then a big dip below the healthy level in the blood. And whole grains contribute an even greater amount of polyphenolics than fresh fruits or vegetables. Also, it is reasonable to realize that the glycemic response of a food can be modified further when it is eaten with a meal. A plentiful supply of polyphenolics from plant foods will keep the glycemic effect of a meal in check.

Bear in mind that a mere excess of 100 calories daily leads to twenty pounds of overweight in ten years (*Parade Magazine,* November 14, 2003, p. 14). Every time you eat refined flour instead of wholegrain flour products, you eat an extra 9 percent in calories. Even more hidden calories are eaten when the refined flour product is an oily bread, a fatty pastry, or is highly sugared. It is better to choose wholegrain products that have no added fat or sugar, and to add the fatty or sugary items as condiments only to the extent that you are exercising to burn off calories. If you sit at your desk all day, you will need to add substantially less to your basic food than if you are walking the Pacific Crest Trail from end to end in a season. When you talk to people who are hiking all day every day, you discover they have a hard time eating enough food to keep up their energy, and they all lose weight.

These charts show the approximate calorie contributions of plant foods, weight for weight. A rough comparison of the calories in each food can be made if you remember that starch, sugar, and proteins are worth 4 calories per gram, soluble fiber is worth 2 calories per gram, and fats are worth 9 calories per gram. Insoluble fiber and water do not contribute calories.

Plant foods can be grouped into seeds, fruits, and vegetables. The fruits and vegetables are noticeably full of water, which explains why they can be eaten in quantity without worrying that too many calories have been ingested. Seed foods are concentrated and are well dried out. It is interesting to look at the differences between the grains, legumes, nuts, and seeds, and use this knowledge when planning your meals. You need a balanced supply of starch, sugar, protein, and fat, and if you eat whole-plant foods to supply this, you automatically take in a healthy amount of fiber and its associated vitamins, minerals, and polyphenolics.

TABLE A.1 • GRAINS

| | Amaranth |
| Barley |
| Buckwheat groats |
| Corn |
| Millet flour |
| Oatmeal |
| Quinoa |
| Rice, brown |
| Rye flour |
| Sorghum |
| Teff |
| Wheat flour, refined |
| Whole Wheat flour |

0 10 20 30 40 50 60 70 80 90 100

Starch   Sugar   Soluble fiber   Insoluble fiber   Water   Protein   Fat

TABLE A.2 • LEGUMES (DRIED, RAW)

Adzuki beans
Blackeyed peas
Fava beans
Garbanzo beans
Haricots
Lentils
Lima beans
Mung beans
Peanuts
Red kidney beans
Soybeans
Split peas

0 10 20 30 40 50 60 70 80 90 100

Starch · Sugar · Soluble fiber · Insoluble fiber · Water · Protein · Fat

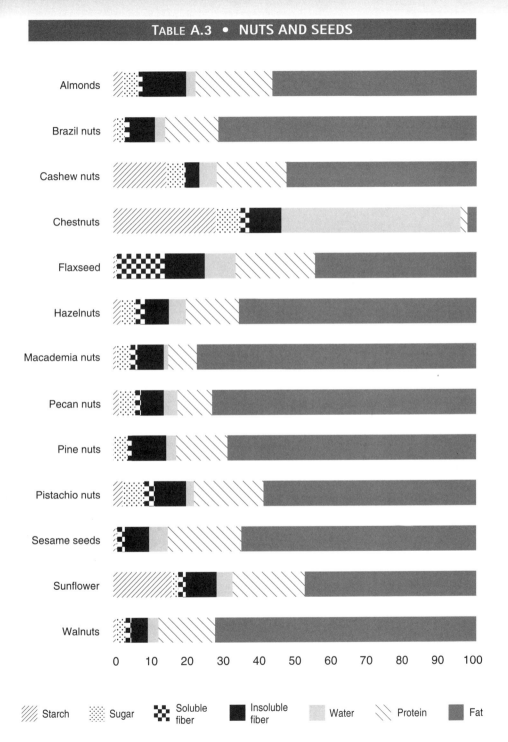

TABLE A.3 • NUTS AND SEEDS

Almonds
Brazil nuts
Cashew nuts
Chestnuts
Flaxseed
Hazelnuts
Macademia nuts
Pecan nuts
Pine nuts
Pistachio nuts
Sesame seeds
Sunflower
Walnuts

0   10   20   30   40   50   60   70   80   90   100

Starch   Sugar   Soluble fiber   Insoluble fiber   Water   Protein   Fat

What's with Fiber?

TABLE A.4 • FRUITS (DRIED, RAW)

Apples

Apricots, fresh

Apricots, dried

Avocado

Bananas

Blackberries

Canteloupe

Cherries

Cranberries

Dates

Figs, fresh

Figs, dried

Grapefruit

Grapes

0   10   20   30   40   50   60   70   80   90   100

Starch   Sugar   Soluble fiber   Insoluble fiber   Water   Protein   Fat

TABLE A.4 (CONT.)   •   FRUITS (DRIED, RAW)

Kiwi

Nectarines

Oranges

Peaches

Pears

Pineapple

Plums

Prunes

Raisins

Raspberries

Strawberries

Tangerines

Watermelon

0   10   20   30   40   50   60   70   80   90   100

/// Starch   Sugar   Soluble fiber   Insoluble fiber   Water   Protein   Fat

TABLE A.5 • VEGETABLES

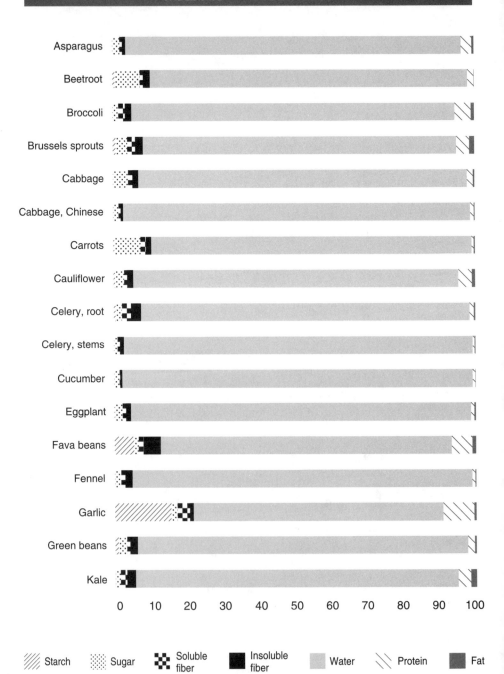

TABLE A.5 (CONT.) • VEGETABLES

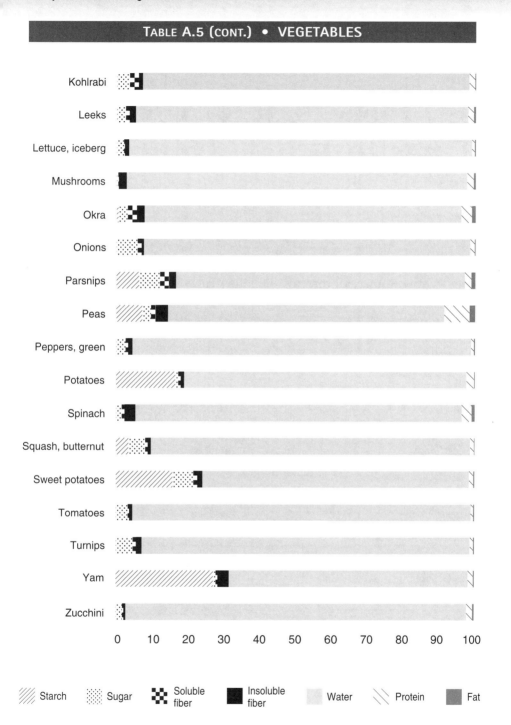

| Starch | Sugar | Soluble fiber | Insoluble fiber | Water | Protein | Fat |

Appendix B

Tables of Total Dietary Fiber in Whole-Plant Foods

The recommended amount of fiber is 30–50 grams per day, according to your height. In your diet, all three of the following whole-plant-food categories should be represented every day.

1. Seed Foods (Grains, Legumes, Nuts, and Seeds)

2. Fruits

3. Vegetables

TABLE B.1. SEED FOODS (GRAINS, LEGUMES, NUTS, AND SEEDS)		
Whole-Plant Foods (Seed Foods)	Serving Size (grams)	Total Dietary Fiber (grams)
GRAINS (Measured Dry)		
Amaranth	1/4 cup (45)	5
Barley	1/4 cup (45)	7
Buckwheat, wholegrain	1 cup (170)	17
Cornmeal, whole ground	1 cup (122)	9
Millet, cooked	1 cup (240)	3
Oatmeal, cooked	1/2 cup (120)	2
Quinoa	1/4 cup (45)	3
Rice, brown, cooked	1 cup (195)	4
Rye flour	1 cup (102)	15
Sorghum	1/4 cup (45)	6
Spaghetti pasta, whole wheat, cooked	1 cup (140)	6
Teff	1/4 cup (45)	6

Whole-Plant Foods (Seed Foods)	Serving Size (grams)	Total Dietary Fiber (grams)
GRAINS (Measured Dry) cont.		
Wheat flour, white	1 cup (125)	3
Wheat flour, wholemeal	1 cup (120)	15
LEGUMES (Cooked)		
Black beans	$\frac{1}{2}$ cup (86)	7
Black-eyed peas	$\frac{1}{2}$ cup (86)	6
Garbanzo beans	$\frac{1}{2}$ cup (82)	6
Great Northern beans	$\frac{1}{2}$ cup (88)	6
Lentils	$\frac{1}{2}$ cup (99)	8
Lima beans	$\frac{1}{2}$ cup (94)	7
Navy beans	$\frac{1}{2}$ cup (91)	6
Peanut butter	2 tablespoons (32)	2
Pinto beans	$\frac{1}{2}$ cup (85)	7
Red kidney beans	$\frac{1}{2}$ cup (88)	6.5
Red Mexican beans	$\frac{1}{2}$ cup (112)	9
Soybeans	$\frac{1}{2}$ cup (86)	5
Split peas	$\frac{1}{2}$ cup (98)	8
NUTS and SEEDS (Dry)		
Almonds, dry roasted	1 oz (28)	4
Brazil nuts	1 oz (28)	1.5
Cashew nuts, dry roasted	1 oz (28)	1
Flaxseeds	1 tablespoon (28)	7
Hazelnuts	1 oz (28)	2.5
Macadamia nuts, salted	1 oz (28)	2.5
Pecan nuts	1 oz (28)	2.5
Pine nuts	1 oz (28)	3
Pistachio nuts, shelled	1 oz (28)	3
Sesame seeds	1 tablespoon (8)	1
Sunflower seeds, dry roasted	1 oz (28)	2.5
Tahini paste	2 tablespoons (30)	2
Walnuts	1 oz (28)	2

Fruits	Serving Size (grams)	Total Dietary Fiber (grams)
TABLE B.2. FRUITS		
FRUITS (Fresh and Dried)		
Apples, with peel	1 apple (138)	4
Apricots, fresh, no pits	3 apricots (105)	3
Apricots, dried	10 halves (35)	9
Avocado (Haas), peeled	1 avocado (173)	8
Banana, peeled	1 banana (118)	3
Blackberries	1 cup (144)	8
Blueberries	1 cup (145)	4
Cantaloupe	1 cup (160)	1.5
Cherries, sweet, red	10 cherries (68)	2
Dates, no pit	10 dates (83)	6
Figs, fresh	2 figs (100)	3.5
Figs, dried	5 figs (80)	9
Grapefruit, pink, peeled	1/2 grapefruit (123)	2
Grapes, red or green, seedless	1 cup (160)	1.5
Kiwi fruit, peeled	1 kiwi (76)	3
Mango, peeled	1 mango (207)	4
Nectarines, no pit	1 nectarine (136)	2
Oranges, peeled, no seeds	1 orange (130)	3
Papaya, no seeds or skin	1 papaya (304)	5
Peaches, peeled, no pit	1 peach (98)	2
Pears, with peel	1 pear (166)	4
Pineapple	1 cup (155)	2
Plums	1 plum (66)	1.5
Prunes, pitted	10 prunes (84)	1.5
Raisins, seedless	1 packet (42)	2
Raspberries	1 cup (123)	8
Strawberries	1 cup (144)	3
Tangerines, peeled, no seeds	1 tangerine (84)	2
Watermelon, no rind or seeds	1 cup (152)	1

	TABLE B.3. VEGETABLES	
Vegetables	Serving Size (grams)	Total Dietary Fiber (grams)
VEGETABLES (Fresh and Canned)		
Artichokes, globe, cooked	1 artichoke (120)	6
Artichokes, Jerusalem, raw	1 cup (150)	2
Asparagus, spears, cooked	4 spears (60)	1
Beets, cooked	$\frac{1}{2}$ cup (85)	2
Broccoli, cooked	$\frac{1}{2}$ cup (78)	2
Brussels sprouts, cooked	$\frac{1}{2}$ cup (78)	2
Cabbage, common varieties, raw	1 cup (70)	2
Cabbage, common varieties, cooked	$\frac{1}{2}$ cup (75)	1.5
Cabbage, Chinese, cooked	$\frac{1}{2}$ cup (60)	1
Carrots, raw	1 carrot (72)	2
Carrots, cooked	$\frac{1}{2}$ cup (78)	3
Cauliflower flowerets, cooked	$\frac{1}{2}$ cup (62)	2
Celery root, cooked	$\frac{1}{2}$ cup (78)	1
Celery, stalks, raw	1 stalk (40)	1
Chard, Swiss, cooked	$\frac{1}{2}$ cup (78)	2
Collard greens, cooked	$\frac{1}{2}$ cup (95)	3
Cucumber, with peel	1 cup (104)	0.5
Eggplant, cooked	$\frac{1}{2}$ cup (50)	1
Escarole/curly endive, raw	1 cup (50)	2
Green beans/string beans, cooked	$\frac{1}{2}$ cup (63)	2
Kale, cooked	$\frac{1}{2}$ cup (65)	1.5
Kohlrabi, raw	1 cup (135)	5
Kohlrabi, cooked	$\frac{1}{2}$ cup (83)	1
Leeks, cooked	$\frac{1}{2}$ cup (52)	0.5
Lettuce, iceberg	1 cup (55)	1
Lettuce, romaine	1 cup (60)	2
Mushrooms, cooked	$\frac{1}{2}$ cup (78)	2
Mustard greens, cooked	$\frac{1}{2}$ cup (70)	1
Okra, cooked	$\frac{1}{2}$ cup (80)	2

Vegetables	Serving Size (grams)	Total Dietary Fiber (grams)
VEGETABLES (Fresh and Canned)		
Onions, cooked	$1/_2$ cup (105)	1
Onions, spring, raw	1 cup (100)	2
Parsnips, cooked	$1/_2$ cup (78)	3
Peas, cooked from frozen	$1/_2$ cup (85)	5
Peas, edible pods, cooked	$1/_2$ cup (80)	2
Peppers, sweet, red or green, raw	1 cup (75)	1
Peppers, sweet, red or green, cooked	$1/_2$ cup (68)	1
Potatoes, baked, with skin	1 potato (202)	5
Potatoes, baked, flesh only	1 potato (156)	2
Rutabaga, cooked	$1/_2$ cup (85)	2
Spinach, raw	1 cup (56)	2
Spinach, cooked	$1/_2$ cup (90)	2
Squash, butternut, baked	$1/_2$ cup (103)	3
Sweet potatoes, baked in skin, peeled	1 potato (114)	3
Tomatoes, raw	1 cup (180)	2
Tomatoes, cooked	$1/_2$ cup (120)	1
Tomatoes, canned	$1/_2$ cup (120)	1
Turnips, cooked	$1/_2$ cup (78)	3
Water chestnuts, canned,	$1/_2$ cup (70)	2
Zucchini, cooked	$1/_2$ cup (90)	1

1) USDA National Database for Standard Reference, Release 16.

2) Table of Food Composition. Main source: USDA National Database for Standard Reference, Release 12, surveys and provisional data, both published and unpublished. In: Whitney, EN, Rolfes, SR. Understanding Nutrition, 8th Ed. Belmont, CA: Wadsworth Publishing, 1999.

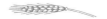

Glossary

Acetic acid. An acid found in vinegar. Also known as a short-chain fatty acid (*see* Short-chain fatty acids) because of its chemical structure.

Anasazi. Ancient Native American people of the southwestern United States.

Antioxidant. A substance, such as vitamin E, selenium, the polyphenol quercetin, and many other organic or inorganic compounds capable of counteracting oxidative damage in the body.

Artery. Any of the small and large blood vessels that carry oxygen and nutrients to all parts of the body.

Atherogenic. Causes formation of plaque in the arteries.

Atherosclerosis. Deposits in the arteries characterized by plaques containing cholesterol in the inner layers of artery walls.

Barm. Celtic word for sourdough (*see* Sourdough) starter. Old recipes (before 1900) for barm include malt, and have a mashing step comparable with beer-making.

Bile acid. Liver-generated steroid acids that commonly occur in the bile and are made from cholesterol.

Blood cholesterol. A fatlike substance produced by the liver and found in animal foods, especially in the fat portion of these foods. It is an important building block of cells and a precursor of various hormones.

Blood sugar. (*See* Glucose.)

Blood sugar, fasting. A laboratory measurement of the concentration of glucose in the blood.

Bowel. The intestines.

Butyric acid. An acid found as part of butter fat. It is also known as a short-chain fatty acid because of its chemical structure.

Cancer, colon. Malignant cells that invade the colon.

Cancer, colorectal. Malignant cells in both the colon and rectum.

Cancer, rectal. Malignant cells that invade the rectum, the last part of the large bowel following the colon.

Carbohydrates, refined. When whole-plant foods (for example, grains), are processed and separated into fractions of digestible carbohydrates, such as white flour (mostly starch), they are called refined carbohydrates. Other examples of refined carbohydrates are white sugar (sucrose) separated from sugar cane juice, and high-fructose corn syrup which is obtained by processing and extracting corn.

Carbohydrates, simple. The simple carbohydrates are built from just one or two sugar molecules (units), for example, glucose, fructose, sucrose.

Cardiovascular disease. (*See* Coronary heart disease.)

Cholesterol. (*See* Blood cholesterol.)

Cholesterol, HDL. (*See* HDL, high-density lipoprotein.)

Cholesterol, LDL. (*See* LDL, low-density lipoprotein.)

Colon. That part of the large intestine extending from the end of the small intestines to the rectum.

Colon cancer. (*See* Cancer, colon.)

Colorectal cancer. (*See* Cancer, colorectal.)

Constipation. Difficult, incomplete, or infrequent evacuation of dry, hardened stool (feces) from the bowels. Transit time for food in the body takes more than two days.

Coprolites. Ancient dried stools found by archeologists in excavations.

Coronary arteries. The arteries that feed and bring oxygen to the heart muscle where clogging leads to heart disease.

Coronary artery disease. (*See* Coronary heart disease.)

Coronary heart disease (CHD). One of the common forms of heart disease where the coronary arteries that feed the heart muscle to give it oxygen and nutrients for its daily work become clogged with cholesterol deposits and can eventually become blocked.

Cotyledons. Leaflike food-storage units in legume seeds (peas and beans).

Crude fiber. (*See* Fiber, crude.)

DASH diet. Dietary approaches to stop hypertension.

Diabetes. Any of several metabolic disorders marked by excessive discharge of urine and persistent thirst, especially one of the two types of diabetes mellitus.

Diabetes, insulin-dependent. (*See* Diabetes, type-1.)

Diabetes, non-insulin-dependent. (*See* Diabetes, type-2.)

Diabetes, type-1. A severe, chronic form of diabetes mellitus caused by insufficient production of insulin and resulting in abnormal metabolism of carbohydrates, fats, and proteins. Typically appearing in childhood or adolescence, the disease is characterized by increased sugar levels in the blood and urine, excessive thirst, frequent urination, acidosis, and wasting. Also called juvenile or insulin-dependent diabetes.

Diabetes, type-2. A mild form of diabetes mellitus that typically appears first in adulthood and is aggravated by obesity and an inactive lifestyle. This disease often has no symptoms, is usually diagnosed by tests that indicate glucose intolerance, and is treated with changes in diet and an exercise regimen. Also called adult-onset or non-insulin-dependent diabetes.

Dietary fiber. (*See* Fiber, dietary.)

Digestive system. Extending from the mouth and including the pharynx, esophagus, stomach, intestines, and digestive glands, this integrated system is responsible for the ingestion, digestion, and absorption of food, and the elimination of wastes from the body at the anus. Also called digestive tract.

Diverticula. Pouches or sacs branching out from a hollow organ or structure, such as the intestine. (The plural of diverticulum.)

Diverticular disease. A condition characterized by the presence of numerous diverticula in the colon. Called diverticulitis when inflammation of a diverticulum or diverticula is present in the intestinal tract, causing fecal (stool) stagnation and pain.

Epidemiological. Studies of health-related states conducted in specific populations of humans. Results of these types of studies are used to help control health problems. They are also called population studies, or observational studies.

Fiber, crude. An old method of fiber analysis that tested only for a small portion of the total fiber. It may be found on some old food labels, but is not in use any longer.

Fiber, dietary. The total fiber in food as found on nutritional labels. It includes both soluble and insoluble fibers.

Free radicals. Unpaired electrons that roam the body causing oxidative damage that can result in degenerative diseases.

Glucose. The principal circulating sugar in the blood and the major energy source of the body.

Gram (g). A metric unit of mass equal to one thousandth of a kilogram; 28.35 grams equal 1 ounce.

Groats. The general term for a whole seed with the inedible husk, hull or shell removed (for example, oat groats or buckwheat groats).

Hemicelluloses. Polymers from mixed sugar units that are part of plant cell walls. Some act as soluble fiber and some as insoluble fiber.

HDL (high-density lipoprotein). A globule that carries cholesterol in the blood. When cholesterol is in this form, it is considered protective, and is often called good cholesterol.

Hypothesis. A premise from which a conclusion is drawn.

Injera. A flat, pancake-like bread made from the small grain teff, a staple food of Ethiopia, cooked on a flat, hot rock in ancient times, and on a griddle today.

Insulin. A hormone that regulates the metabolism of carbohydrates and fats, especially the conversion of glucose to glycogen, which lowers the blood glucose level.

Intestines, large. The portion of the intestine that extends from the end of the small intestine to the anus, forming an arch around the folds and coils of the small intestine and including the cecum (the large blind pouch forming the beginning of the large intestine), colon, rectum, and anal canal.

Intestines, small. The winding, upper part of the intestine where digestion takes place and nutrients are absorbed by the blood.

Large intestines. (*See* Intestines, large.)

LDL (low-density lipoprotein). One of the globules that carries cholesterol in the blood. When cholesterol is in this form, it is considered much more damaging and causes bad deposits (plaques) in the arteries that slowly narrow the openings of the blood vessels. That is why LDL is often called bad cholesterol.

Lipoproteins. A term derived, from *lipo,* which means fat, and protein. There are many large particles, or globules, and they are composed of fats, proteins, and related compounds that contain cholesterol and carry it around in the blood. There are many of them with many different fractions. The two most commonly used in determining whether to be concerned about cholesterol levels are low-density lipoprotein (LDL) and high-density lipoprotein (HDL).

Malt, malted grain. When whole grains are sprouted and then dried, the product is a *malted* grain. Enzymes, including amylases and phytases, which are increased on sprouting the grain, remain in the malt if it is dried at room temperature. Roasting at higher temperatures, to produce dark malt, usually destroys the enzyme activity.

Masa. Flour for tortillas made from ground nixtamal.

Mash, mashing. Any process in which malt enzymes are allowed to work on grains in the presence of adequate moisture and optimal temperatures. Many of the grain components are modified—for example, starch is broken down into oligosaccharides and simple sugars, phytonutrients and minerals are released.

Nixtamal. Corn product resulting from treatment with lime, which releases the niacin; used in making tortillas.

Oatmeal. *Old meaning:* Whole oats (groats) that have been ground to a flour (meal), coarse or fine; this is currently a rare product. *Modern meaning:* Rolled oats, or whole oat (groat) flakes. (*See* Groats.)

Oligosaccharides. Intermediate-length polysaccharides, or chains of two to twenty sugar molecules.

ORAC. Oxygen radical absorbance capacity.

Petroglyph. A carving or line drawing on rock made by prehistoric people.

Phenolics. A broad group of related compounds commonly found in plants; they are colored shades of brown, red, and purple, and are antioxidants. Often several phenolics are linked in chains (polyphenolics), as, for example, with bioflavonoids in fruits or resveratrol in grapes.

Phenols. Alternative name for phenolics.

Phytates. Compounds related to phytic acid (inositol hexa-phosphoric acid) commonly found in seeds. They have the property of binding minerals, unless broken down by the enzyme phytase, which is activated when seeds are soaked or sprouted. Phytates are protective against colon cancer.

Phytochemicals. Beneficial chemical compounds found in plant foods (*Phyto* means plant in Greek.) Although it is now known that many of these compounds are important to good health, they were not considered beneficial until recently.

Plant sterols. Compounds contained in plant foods that are somewhat similar in their chemical structure to cholesterol, but which actually help to lower blood cholesterol and may possibly have a protective effect against colon cancer.

Plaques. Deposits of cholesterol and fibers in the inner wall of arteries.

Polenta. Cornmeal and water cooked until it becomes thick. Salt, cheese and other flavorings are added. It is served in a dish after it has set until firm. Sometimes it is further baked.

Polymer. Molecules of one or two kinds, strongly linked together in a chain. The polymer has totally different properties compared with the contributing molecules—cellulose is a polymer of glucose, for example.

Polyphenols. A polymer of phenolic compounds (*see* Polymer and Phenolics).

Porridge. Historical word used in Britain for hot-cereal dish made from wholegrain flour and boiling water. Proportions of water to flour, vary from 1 to 2 parts of water for each part of flour. Essentially the grain starch becomes gelatinized as a result of the addition of hot water.

Propionic acid. A short-chain fatty acid, produced as a result of fermentation (during cheesemaking, for example).

Rectal cancer. (*See* Cancer, rectal.)

Rectum. The terminal portion of the large intestine, extending from the sigmoid flexure (an S-shaped section of the colon between the descending section and the rectum, also called the sigmoid colon) to the anal canal.

Reductionism. Attempting to find just one or two causes for a complex problem. Reducing findings to fit a single theory.

Refined carbohydrates. (*See* Carbohydrates, refined.)

Resistant starch. A product formed in starchy foods during cooking that resists the digestive enzymes in the body, although it can be digested by the intestinal bacteria.

Short-chain fatty acids. Acid component of fats, with a characteristic structure consisting of a chain of carbon atoms. The smallest examples—acetic, butyric, and propionic acids—are called short-chain fatty acids.

Simple carbohydrates. (*See* Carbohydrates, simple.)

Small intestines. (*See* Intestines, small.)

Sourdough. A fermented mixture of flour and water containing compatible yeasts and lactic bacteria that is used to leaven breads. The sourness is due to the acids produced by the lactic bacteria.

Tartaric acid. An acid found in reasonable amounts in grapes and their products—raisins, wine, grape juice, especially when unfiltered, and in the tropical and semitropical tamarind fruit, and the products of these fruits.

Total blood cholesterol. The sum of the cholesterol in all types of lipoproteins (HDL, LDL, VLDL). Scientists say plasma or serum cholesterol, meaning the cholesterol in the plasma or serum (the blood after the red cells and white cells have been removed).

Transit time. The time taken by food to travel through the body, from the time it is eaten to the time the residue is excreted in the stool. One to two days is optimal.

Triglycerides. One of the ways fats are found in foods and in the body. The fats are built from glycerol and fatty acids. The glycerol can join with one (monoglyceride) to three fatty acids (triglycerides). Used by the body for energy.

Wholemeal. Wholegrain flour obtained by milling a whole grain, such as wheat, and collecting the total product without removing or adding anything.

Resources

Vegetables, Fruits, and Nuts

The following resources are for farmers' markets, community-supported agriculture projects (CSAs), and stores selling local and regional produce.

Local Chambers of Commerce

Where are the closest farmers' markets? This can usually be answered by your local Chamber of Commerce. It's well worth asking because at farmers' markets you will have the opportunity of buying directly from farmers who grow your fruits, grains, nuts, seeds, and vegetables. Usually the markets are seasonal, outdoors, and open for half a day or an evening each week.

Local Newspapers

Articles on locally produced vegetables and fruits in season are popular topics in local newspapers. These provide a good lead to finding interesting local farms that sell directly to farm visitors, or farms that offer a community-supported agriculture (CSA) opportunity. In a CSA, the farmer usually provides a basket of selected produce from the farm each week during the growing season. Members pay the farmer ahead of time for a season of produce, giving the farmer the benefits of predictable income.

Biodynamic Farming and Gardening Association, Inc.
25844 Butler Road
Junction City, OR 97448
Ph: 541-998-0105/888-516-7797
Fax: 541-998-0106
Website: www.biodynamics.com
e-mail: biodynamic@aol.com
Website lists CSA farmers by state.

California Certified Organic Farmers

1115 Mission Street
Santa Cruz, CA 95060-3526
Ph: 831-423-2263
Fax: 831-423-4528
Website: www.ccof.org
e-mail: ccof@ccof.org
Annual directory of organic farmers and their products.

Local Harvest

220 21st Avenue
Santa Cruz, CA 95062
Ph: 831-475-8150
Website: www.localharvest.org
e-mail: info@localharvest.org
List of local farmers' markets, local farms, and CSAs.

The New Farm

The Rodale Institute
611 Siegfriedale Road
Kutztown, PA 19530
Ph: 610-683-1400
Fax: 610-683-8548
Website: www.newfarm.org
e-mail: info@newfarm.org

"Farmer-to-farmer know-how from the Rodale Institute." This is a list of local farmers who farm and sell directly to the public at farmers' markets through CSAs.

Oregon Tilth, Inc.

470 Lancaster Drive NE
Salem, OR 97301
Ph: 503-378-0690
Fax: 503-378-0809
Website: www.tilth.org
e-mail: organic@tilth.org
Annual directory of growers and products.

Whole Foods Market

550 Bowie Street
Austin, TX 78703-4677
Ph: 512-477-4455
Fax: 512-482-7000
Website: www.wholefoods.com
e-mail: info@wholefoods.com
Chain of supermarkets that specialize in providing an abundant selection of fresh, largely organic, produce; some selections are local.

Whole Grains, Legumes, and Seeds

Most of these vendors have a line of organic products, but be sure to ask for 100-percent whole grains, as some also sell refined grains.

Arrowhead Mills

The Hain Celestial Group
4600 Sleepytime Drive
Boulder, CO 80301

Ph: 800-434-4246
Website: www.arrowheadmills.com
e-mail: llehndor@hain-celestial.com
Stone-ground flours, grains, and beans.

Bob's Red Mill
5209 SE International Way
Milwaukie, OR 97222
Ph: 800-349-2173
Fax: 503-653-1339
Website: www.bobsredmill.com
e-mail: info@bobsredmill.com
Stone-ground flours, grains, beans, and seeds.

Briess Malt and Ingredients Company
625 South Irish Road
Chilton, WI 53014-0229
Ph: 920-849-7711
Fax: 920-849-4277
Website: www.briess.com
e-mail: info@briess.com
Malted barley, rye, and wheat.

Giusto's Specialty Foods
344 Littlefield Road
South San Francisco, CA 94080
Ph: 650-873-6566
Fax: 650-873-2826
Website: www.giustos.com
e-mail: info@worldpantry.com
Stone-ground flours, grains, beans, and seeds.

The Grain Place
1904 North Highway 14
Marquette, NE 68854
Ph: 402-854-2566
Fax: 402-854-2566
Grains, including hull-less barley, and seeds.

Hodgson Mill, Inc.
1203 Niccum Avenue
Effingham, IL 62401
Ph: 800-347-0105
Fax: 217-347-0198
Website: www.hodgsonmill.com
e-mail: CustomerService@Hodgson Mill.com
Stone-ground wholegrain cereals, flours, pasta, and seeds.

Inca Organics
PO Box 61-8154
Chicago, IL 60661
Ph: 312-575-9880
Fax: 312-575-9881
Website: www.incaorganics.com
e-mail: incaorganics@aol.com
Quinoa and amaranth.

The Kamut Association
333 Kamut Lane
Big Sandy, MT 59520-8218
Ph: 406-378-3105
Fax: 406-378-3106
Website: www.kamut.com
e-mail: bob.quinn@kamut.com
Kamut product information.

Lundberg Family Farms
5370 Church Street
Richvale, CA 95974
Ph: 530-882-4551
Fax: 530-882-4500
Website: www.lundberg.com
e-mail: info@lundberg.com
Brown rice varieties.

Montana Flour and Grains
2500 Chouteau Street
Fort Benton, MT 59442
Ph: 406-622-5436
Fax: 406-622-5439
Website: www.montanaflour.com
e-mail: info@montanaflour.com
Kamut and wheat.

Purity Foods
2871 West Jolly Road
Okemos, MI 48864
Ph: 517-351-9231
Fax: 517-351-9391
Website: www.purityfoods.com
e-mail: info@purityfoods.com
Spelt wheat.

The Teff Company
PO Box A
Caldwell, ID 83606
Ph: 888-822-2221

Website: www.teffco.com
e-mail: info@teffco.com
Teff flour and grain.

Wheat Montana Farms and Bakery
10778 Highway 287
Three Forks, MT 59752
Ph: 406-285-3614/800-535-2798
Fax: 406-285-3749
Website: www.wheatmontana.com
e-mail: info@wheatmontana.com
Wheat flour and grain.

White Mountain Farm
5305 North Highway 17
Mosca, CO 81146
Ph: 800-364-3019
Fax: 719-378-2897
Website: www.whitemountainfarm.com
e-mail: paul@whitemountainfarm.com
Quinoa.

Mushrooms and Sea Vegetation

Far West Fungi
1 Ferry Building, Shop 34
San Francisco, CA 94111
Ph: 415-989-9090
Fax: 415-989-9090
Website: www.farwestfungi.com
e-mail: imgarrone@hotmail.com
Wild and cultivated mushrooms.

Fungi Perfecti
PO Box 7634
Olympia, WA 98507
Ph: 360-426-9292/800-780-9126
Fax: 360-426-9377

Website: www.fungiperfecti.com
e-mail: mycomedia@aol.com
Edible and medicinal mushroom-growing kits.

Gourmet Mushrooms, Inc.
2901 Gravenstein Highway North
Sebastopol, CA 95472
Ph: 707-823-1743
Fax: 707-823-1507
Website: www.mycopia.com
e-mail: info@gourmetmushroomsinc.com
Wild and cultivated mushrooms.

Maine Coast Sea Vegetables
3 Georges Pond Road
Franklin, ME 04634
Ph: 207-565-2907
Fax: 207-565-2144
Website: www.seaveg.com
e-mail: info@seaveg.com
Seaweeds.

Rising Tide Sea Vegetables
PO Box 1914
Mendocino, CA 95460
Ph: 707-964-5663
Fax: 707-962-0599
Website: www.loveseaweed.com
e-mail: risingtide@mcn.org
Seaweeds.

Starters for Wholegrain Breads and Soybean Products

Alton Spiller, Inc.
PO Box 696
Los Altos, CA 94023
Ph: 650-941-8288
Fax: 650-948-8540
Website: www.barmbaker.com
e-mail: barmbaker@aol.com
Barm bread starters.

G.E.M. Cultures
30301 Sherwood Road
Fort Bragg, CA 95437
Ph: 707-964-2922
Website: www.gemcultures.com
Sourdough starters, soy cultures, and tofu form kits.

Growing Your Own Vegetables—Seeds and Supplies

**Ecology Action and Bountiful
  Gardens Seed Catalog**
18001 Shafer Ranch Road
Willits, CA 95490-9626
Ph: 707-459-6410
Fax: 707-459-1925
Website: www.bountifulgardens.org
e-mail: bountiful@sonic.net
Vegetable seeds and books.

Seed Savers Exchange
3094 North Winn Road
Decorah, IA 52101
Ph: 563-382-5990
Fax: 563-382-5872
Website: www.seedsavers.org

e-mail for *membership info*:
steph@seedsavers.org
e-mail for *ordering and shipping*:
tara@seedsavers.org *or*
kathy@seedsavers.org
Vegetable-seed savers exchange catalog.

The Cook's Garden
PO Box C5030
Warminster, PA 18974
Ph: 800-457-9703
Fax: 800-457-9705
Website: www.cooksgarden.com
e-mail: cooksgarden@earthlink.net
Vegetable seeds.

Plant Food Information

Sphera
PO Box 338
Los Altos, CA 94023-0338
Ph: 650-941-7251
Fax: 650-948-8540
Website: www.sphera.org
e-mail: spiller@sphera.org
Videos and books.

U.S. National Library of Medicine
8600 Rockville Pike
Bethesda, MD 20894
Website: www.PubMed.gov
Abstracts of research papers are freely accessible at this website; it is possible to enter key words from your questions that will lead you to the relevant abstracts.

Whole Grain Connection
PO Box 696
Los Altos, CA 94023
Ph: 650-941-8288
Fax: 650-948-8540
Website: www.sustainablegrains.org
e-mail: barmbaker@aol.com
Newsletter, old-fashioned wheat-seed catalog.

References

BOOKS

Alford, J, Duguid, N. *Flatbreads and Flavors.* New York, NY: William Morrow and Company, Inc., 1995.

Allinson, Thomas. *Advantages of Wholemeal Bread.* London, England: London Echo, 1888.

Atwood, M. *Adventures in Indian Cooking.* Bombay, India: JAICO Publishing, 1969.

Barash, CW. *Edible Flowers.* Golden, CO: Fulcrum Publishing, 1994.

Blumenthal, M. *The ABC Clinical Guide to Herbs.* Austin, TX: The American Botanical Council, 2003.

Board on Science and Technology for International Development, National Research Council. *Lost Crops of Africa, Vol. 1: Grains.* Washington, DC: National Academy Press, 1996.

Brodribb, AJM. "Dietary fiber in diverticular disease of the colon" in *Medical Aspects of Dietary Fiber.* Spiller, GA, Kay, RM. (eds.) New York, NY: Plenum Medical Book Company, 1980.

Burkitt DP, Trowell, HC. *Refined Carbohydrate Foods and Disease—Some Implications of Dietary Fibre.* London, England: Academic Press, 1975.

Burne, J. *Treatise on the Causes and Consequences of Constipation.* New Orleans, LA: Haswell, Barrington and Haswell, 1840.

Bushuk, W. *Rye: Production, Chemistry and Technology.* St. Paul, MN: American Association of Cereal Chemists, 2001.

Carper, J. *Miracle Cures.* New York, NY: Harper Collins, 1997.

Carr, D. *The Necessity of Brown Bread for Digestion, Nourishment and Sound Health and the Injurious Effects of White Bread.* London, England: Effingham Wilson, 1847.

Cleave, TL. *The Saccharine Disease.* New Canaan, CT: Keats Publishing, Inc., 1975.

Davidson, A. *The Oxford Companion to Food.* Oxford, England: Oxford University Press, 1999.

Davidson, SR, Passmore, R, Brock, JD, et al. *Human Nutrition and Dietetics* (6th Ed). New York, NY: Churchill Livingstone, 1975.

Dendy, DAV. (ed.) *Sorghum and Millets: Chemistry and Technology.* St. Paul, MN: American Association of Cereal Chemists, 1995.

Dietary Fiber. Proceedings of the Miles Symposium '76, presented by The Nutrition Society of Canada. June 14, 1976. Dalhousie University, Halifax, Nova Scotia.

Dirar, HA. *The Indigenous Fermented Foods of the Sudan.* Wallingford, England: CAB International, 1993.

Evans, O. *The Young Mill-Wright and Miller's Guide,* 1795. (Reprinted from the 1st Ed. Wallingford, PA: Oliver Evans Press, 1990.)

Fabricant, F. *Elizabeth Berry's Great Bean Book.* Berkeley, CA: Ten Speed Press, 1999.

Farquhar, JW, Spiller, GA. *Diagnosis: Heart Disease.* New York, NY: W.W. Norton, 2001.

Fitzgibbon, T. *A Taste of Ireland in Food and Pictures.* London, England: Pan Books, 1968.

Goodhart, RS, Shils, ME. *Modern Nutrition in Health and Disease* (6th Ed). Philadelphia, PA: Lea and Febiger, 1980.

Graham, S. *Treatise on Bread and Bread Making,* Boston, MA: Light and Stearns, 1837. (Reprinted: Payson, AZ: Leaves-of-Autumn Books, 1991.)

Ho, CT, Lee, CY, Huang, MT. (eds.) *Phenolic Compounds in Food and Their Effects on Health.* ACS Symposium Series 506. Washington, DC: American Chemical Society, 1992.

Holland, B, Unwin, ID, Buss, BH. *McCance and Widdowson's The Composition of Food.* Supplements: *Cereals and Cereal Products* (4th Ed.), *Vegetables, Herbs and Spices* (4th Ed.), *Fruit and Nuts* (5th Ed.). London, England: Royal Society of Chemistry/Ministry of Agriculture, Fisheries and Food, 1988–1992.

Jago, W, Jago, WC. *The Technology of Bread-Making.* Chicago, IL: Baker's Helper Company, 1911.

Jones, E. *American Food.* New York, NY: E.P. Dutton and Co., 1975.

Joseph, JA, Nadeau, DA, Underwood, A. *The Color Code.* New York, NY: Hyperion, 2002.

Juliano, BO. (ed.) *Rice: Chemistry and Technology.* St. Paul, MN: American Association of Cereal Chemists, 1985.

Kellogg, JH. *Colon Hygiene.* Battle Creek, MI: The Modern Medicine Publishing Company, 1927. (Revised Edition.)

Kiple, KF, Ornelas, KC. (eds.) *The Cambridge World History of Food,* Vols. I and II. Cambridge, England: Cambridge University Press, 2000.

Kiritsakis, AK. (ed.) *Olive Oil.* Champaign, Illinois: American Oil Chemists Society, 1990.

Kliks, M. "Paleo-dietetics: a review of the role of dietary fiber in pre-agricultural human diets" in *Topics in Dietary Fiber Research.* Spiller, GA, Amen, RJ. (eds.) New York, NY: Plenum Press, 1978.

Kreger-van Rij, NJW. (ed.) *The Yeasts: A Taxonomic Study.* Amsterdam, Netherlands: Elsevier Science Publishers, 1984.

Lappé, FM. *Diet for a Small Planet,* 20th Anniversary Ed. New York, NY: Ballantine Books, 1991.

MacGregor, AW, Bhatty, RS. (eds.) *Barley: Chemistry and Technology.* St. Paul, MN: American Association of Cereal Chemists, 1993.

Marquart, L, Slavin JL, Fulcher, RG. (eds.) *Whole Grain Foods in Health and Disease.* St. Paul, MN: American Association of Cereal Chemists, 2002.

Mazza, G, Miniati, E. *Anthocyanins in Fruits, Grains and Vegetables.* Boca Raton, FL: CRC Press, 1993.

McCarrison R. *Studies in Deficiency Disease.* London, England: Henry Frowde and Hodder and Stoughton, 1921.

McNeill, FM. *The Scots Kitchen.* London, England: Blackie and Sons, 1929.

Merck Index, The (11th Ed). Rahway, NJ: Merck and Co., 1989.

Mesfin, DJ. *Exotic Ethiopian Cooking.* Falls Church, VA: Ethiopian Cookbook Enterprises, 1990.

Morris, DH. *Flax: A Health and Nutrition Primer.* Winnipeg, Canada: Flax Council of Canada, 2003.

National Research Council. *Lost Crops of the Incas.* Washington, DC: National Academy Press, 1989.

Ojakangas, B. *The Great Scandinavian Baking Book.* Boston, MA: Little, Brown and Company, 1988.

Owen, S. *The Rice Book.* New York, NY: St. Martin's Press, 1994.

Price, WA. *Nutrition and Physical Degeneration: A Comparison of Primitive and Modern Diets and Their Effects.* Los Angeles, CA: The American Academy of Applied Nutrition, 1939.

Reddy, NR, Pierson, MD, Sathe, SK, et al. (eds.) *Phytates in Cereals and Legumes.* Boca Raton, FL: CRC Press, 1989.

Rice-Evans, CA, Packer, L. (eds.) *Flavonoids in Health and Disease.* New York, NY: Marcel Dekker, Inc., 1998.

Salminen, S, von Wright, A. (eds.) *Lactic Acid Bacteria* (2nd Ed). New York, NY: Marcel Dekker Inc., 1998.

Spencer, C. *The Vegetable Book.* New York, NY: Rizzoli, 1996.

Spiller, GA. (ed.) *CRC Handbook of Dietary Fiber* (3rd Ed). Boca Raton, FL: CRC Press, 2001.

Spiller, GA. *Healthy Nuts.* Garden City Park, NY: Avery Publishing Group, 2000.

Spiller, GA. (ed.) *The Methylxanthine Beverages and Foods: Chemistry, Consumption and Health Effects.* New York, NY: Alan R. Liss, Inc., 1984.

Spiller, GA. *Topics in Dietary Fiber Research.* New York, NY: Plenum Press, 1978.

Spiller, GA, Amen, RJ. *Fiber in Human Nutrition.* New York, NY: Plenum Press, 1976.

Spiller, GA, Bruce, B. *Cancer Survivor's Nutrition and Health Guide.* Rocklin, CA: Prima Publishing, 1997.

Spiller, GA, Hubbard, R. *The Power of Ancient Foods.* Summertown, TN: Book Publishing Company, 2003.

Spiller, GA, Madison, D. *Eat Your Way to Better Health.* Rocklin, CA: Prima Publishing, 1996.

Steinkraus, KH. (ed.) *Handbook of Indigenous Fermented Foods* (2nd Ed). New York, NY: Marcel Dekker, Inc., 1995.

The Visual Food Encyclopedia. Montreal, Canada: Les Éditions Québec/Amérique, Inc, 1996.

Trowell, HC, Burkitt, DP. *Western Diseases: Their Emergence and Prevention.* Cambridge, MA: Harvard University Press, 1981.

USDA National Nutrient Database for Standard Reference, Release 16. Nutrient Data Laboratory Home Page: www.nal.usda.gov/fnic/foodcomp United States Department of Agriculture, Agricultural Research Service, 2004.

Walker, H. (ed.) Oxford Symposium on Food and Cookery 1989. *Staple Foods.* London, England: Prospect Books, 1990.

Web, Denise. "The Year's Best Food News." *Parade Magazine.* November 14, 2003, p.14.

Webster, FH. (ed.) *Oats: Chemistry and Technology.* St. Paul, MN: American Association of Cereal Chemists, 1986.

Whistler, RL, BeMiller, N. *Industrial Gums.* London, England: Academic Press, 1973.

White, PJ, Johnson, LA. (eds.) *Corn: Chemistry and Technology.* St. Paul, MN: American Association of Cereal Chemists, 1987. (2nd Ed., 2003.)

Whitney, EN, Rolfes, S. *Table of Food Composition, in Understanding Nutrition* (8th Ed). Belmont, CA: Wadsworth Publishing, 1999. (Main source: USDA database, Release 12, surveys, and provisional data both published and unpublished.)

Wilson, AC. *Food and Drink in Britain.* Chicago, IL: Academy Chicago Publishers, 1991.

Wilson, RT. *Let's Do Lunch.* Bonita Springs, FL: Sunshine Publications, Inc., 2003.

CLINICAL STUDIES

Part One

Azar, M, Verette, E, Brun, S. "Comparative study of fresh and fermented bilberry juices—state and modification of the coloring pigments." *Journal of Food Sciences.* 55:164, 1990.

Evans, RC, Fear, S, Ashby, D, et al. "Diet and colorectal cancer: an investigation of the lectin/galactose hypothesis." *Gastroenterology.* 122(7):1784–1792, June 2002.

Scalbert, A, Morand, C, Manach, C. et al. "Absorption and metabolism of polyphenols in the gut and impact on health." *Biomedical Pharmocotherapy.* 56:276–282, 2002.

Part Two

Aldoori, WH, Giovannucci, EL, Rockett, HR, et al. "A prospective study of dietary fiber types and symptomatic diverticular disease in men." *Journal of Nutrition.* 128(4):714–719, April 1998.

Aldoori, WH, Ryan-Harshman, M. "Preventing diverticular disease. Review of recent evidence on high-fibre diets." *Canadian Family Physician.* 48:1632–1637, October 2002.

Alexander, HM, Harris, A, Lockwood, LP, et al. "Risk factors for cardiovascular disease and diabetes in two groups of Hispanic Americans with differing dietary habits." *Journal of the American College of Nutrition.* 18(2):127–136, 1999.

Anderson, JW, Randles, KM, Kendall, CWC, et al. "Carbohydrate and fiber recommendations for individuals with diabetes." *American Journal of Clinical Nutrition.* February, 2004.

Bazzanno, LA, He, J, Loria, C, et al. "Legume consumption and risk of coronary heart disease in US men and women: NHANES I Epidemiologic Follow-up Study." *Archives of Internal Medicine.* 161(21):2573–2578, November 26, 2001.

Bingham, S. "Meat, starch and non-starch polysaccharides: are epidemiological and experimental findings consistent with acquired genetic alterations in sporadic colorectal cancer?" *Cancer Letters.* 114(1–2):25–34, March 19, 1997.

Chen, H, Sheu, WH, Tai,T, et al. "Konjac supplement alleviated hypercholesterolemia and hyperglycemia in type-2 diabetic subjects—a randomized double-blind trial." *Journal of the American College of Nutrition.* 22(1):36–42, 2003.

Cowgill, GR, Anderson, WE. "Laxative effect of wheat bran and washed bran in healthy men." *Journal of the American Medical Association.* 98:1866, 1932.

Cummings, JH, Hill, MJ, Jenkins, DJ, et al. "Changes in fecal composition and colonic function due to cereal fiber." *American Journal of Clinical Nutrition.* 29(12)a:1468–1473, December 1976.

Davy, BM, Melby, CL. "The effect of fiber-rich carbohydrates on features of Syndrome X." *Journal of the American Dietetic Association.* 103(1):86–96, January 2003.

Djoussé, L, Arnett, DK, Coon, H, et al. "Fruit and vegetable consumption and LDL cholesterol: the National Heart, Lung and Blood Institute Family Heart Study." *American Journal of Clinical Nutrition.* 79(2):213–217, 2004.

Evans, DF. "Physicochemical environment of the colon." *European Journal of Cancer Prevention.* 7 Suppl 2:S79–80, May 1998.

Fuchs, CS, Giovannucci, EL, Colditz, GA. "Dietary fiber and the risk of colorectal cancer and adenoma in women." *The New England Journal of Medicine.* 340(3):169–176, 1999.

Gear, JS, Ware, A, Fursdon, P, et al. "Symptomless diverticular disease and intake of dietary fiber." *The Lancet.* 1(8115):511–514. March 10, 1979.

Gerhardt, A, Gallo, NB. "Full-fat rice bran and oat bran similarly reduce hypercholesterolemia in humans." *The Journal of Nutrition.* 28(5): 865–869, May 1998.

Giacco, R, Clemente, G, Riccardi, G. "Dietary fiber in treatment of diabetes: myth or reality?" *Journal of Digestive and Liver Disorders.* 34 Suppl 2:S140–144, September 2002.

Giacosa, A, Hill, MJ, Davies, GJ. "Fibres and colorectal cancer: should we change our dietary advice on prevention?" *Journal of Digestive and Liver Disorders.* 34 Suppl 2:S121–123, September 2002.

Goel, V, Ooraikul, B, Basu, TK. "Cholesterol lowering effect of rhubarb stalk fiber in hypercholesterolemic men." *Journal of the American College of Nutrition.* 16(6): 600–604, December 1997.

Hu, FB, Willett, WC. "Optimal diets for prevention of coronary heart disease." *Journal of the American Medical Association.* 288(20):2569–2578, November 27, 2002.

Jenab, M, Thompson, LU. "The influence of phytic acid in wheat bran on early biomarkers of colon carcinogenesis." *Carcinogenesis.* 19(6):1087–1092, June 1998.

Hill, M. "Dietary fiber and colon cancer: where do we go from here?" *Proceedings of the Nutrition Society.* 62(1):63–65. February 2003.

Hill, MJ. "Mechanisms of diet and colon carcinogenesis." *European Journal of Cancer Prevention.* 8 Suppl 1:S95–98, December 1999.

Jenkins, DJ, Kendall, CW, Augustin, LS, et al. "High complex carbohydrate or lente carbohydrate foods?" *American Journal of Medicine.* 113 Suppl 9B:30S-37S. December 30, 2002.

Jenkins, DJ, Kendall, CW, Marchie, A, et al. "The Garden of Eden—plant based diets, the genetic drive to conserve cholesterol and its implications for heart disease in the 21st century." *Comparative Biochemical Physiology and Molecular Integrated Physiology.* 136(1):141–151, September 2003.

Jenkins, DJ, Kendall, CW, Vuksan, V, et al. "Effect of cocoa bran on low-density lipoprotein oxidation and fecal bulking." *Archives of Internal Medicine.* 160(15):2374–2379, August 14–28, 2000.

Jensen, CD, Haskell, W, Whittam, JH. "Long-term effects of water-soluble dietary fiber in the management of hypercholesterolemia in healthy men and women." *American Journal of Cardiology.* 79(1):34–37, January 1997.

Kalkwarf, HJ, Bell, RC, Khoury, JC, et al. "Dietary fiber intakes and insulin requirements in pregnant women with type-1 diabetes." *Journal of the American Dietetic Association.* 101(3):305–310. March 2001.

La Vecchia, C, Ferraroni, M, Franceschi, S, et al. "Fibers and breast cancer risk." *Nutrition and Cancer.* 28(3):264–269, 1997.

LeMarchand, L, Hankin, JH, Wilkens, LR, et al. "Dietary fiber and colorectal cancer risk." *Epidemiology.* 8(6):658–665, November 1997.

Levi, F, Pasche, C, Lucchini, F, et al. "Dietary fibre and the risk of colorectal cancer." *European Journal of Cancer.* 37(16):2091–2096, November 2001.

Liu, S, Willett, WC, Manson, JE, et al. "Relation between changes in intakes of dietary fiber and grain products and changes in weight and development of obesity among middle-aged women." *American Journal of Clinical Nutrition.* 78:920–927, 2003.

McIntosh, M, Miller, C. "A diet containing food rich in soluble and insoluble fiber improves glycemic control and reduces hyperlipidemia among patients with type-2 diabetes mellitus." *Nutrition Reviews.* 59(2):52–55, February 2001.

McMillan, L, Butcher, SK, Pongracz, J, et al. "Opposing effects of butyrate and bile acids on apoptosis of human colon adenoma cells: differential activation of PKC and MAP kinases." *British Journal of Cancer.* 88:748–753, 2003.

Painter, NS. "Intrasigmoid pressures in diverticulosis of the colon." *British Medical Journal.* 1:309, 1963.

Painter, NS, Burkitt, DP. "Diverticular disease of the colon: a deficiency disease of Western civilization." *British Medical Journal.* 2:450–454, 1971.

Reddy, BS, Hirose, Y, Cohen, LA, et al. "Preventive potential of wheat bran fractions against experimental colon carcinogenesis: implications for human colon cancer prevention." *Cancer Research.* 60(17)a:4792–4797, September 1, 2000.

Rose, G, Blackburn, H, Keys, A, et al. "Colon cancer and blood cholesterol." *The Lancet.* 1(7850):181–183, February 9, 1974.

Scheppach, W, Boxberger, F, Luhrs, H. et al. "Effect of nutrition factors on the pathogenesis of colorectal carcinoma." (article in German). Zentralblatt für Chirurgie. 125 Suppl 1:5–7, 2000.

Slattery, ML, Curtin, KP, Edwards, SL, et al. "Plant foods, fiber, and rectal cancer." *American Journal of Clinical Nutrition.* 79(20):274–281, February 2004.

Spiller, GA, Amen, RJ. Letter: research on dietary fibre. *The Lancet.* 2(7891):1259, November 23,1974.

Spiller, GA, Farquhar, JW, Gates, JE, et al. "Guar gum and plasma cholesterol. Effect of guar gum and an oat fiber source on plasma lipoproteins and cholesterol in hypercholesterolemic adults." *Arteriosclerosis and Thrombosis.* 11(5):12104–12108, September/October 1991.

Spiller, GA, Story, JA, Furomoto, EJ, et al. "Effect of tartaric acid and dietary fibre from sun-dried raisins on colonic function and on bile acid and volatile fatty acid excretion in healthy adults." *British Journal of Nutrition.* 90(4):803–807. October 2003.

Truswell, AS. "Dietary fibre and blood lipids." *Current Opinion in Lipidology.* 6(1):14–19, February 1995.

Wu, H, Dwyer, KM, Fan, Z, et al. "Dietary fiber and progression of atherosclerosis: the Los Angeles Atherosclerosis Study." *American Journal of Clinical Nutrition.* 78(6):1085–1091, December 2003.

PART THREE

Grains, Nuts, Seeds, and Legumes

Cho, S, Dietrich, M, Brown, CJP, et al. "The effect of breakfast type on total daily energy intake and body mass index: results from the Third National Health and Nutrition Examination Survey (NHANES III)." *Journal of the American College of Nutrition.* 22:296, 2003.

Freudenheim, L, Graham, S, Horvath, PJ, et al. "Risks associated with source of fiber and fiber components in cancer of the colon and rectum." *Cancer Research.* 50:3295–3300, 1990.

MacLennan, R, Jenson, OM, Mosbech, J, et al. "Transit time, stool weight, and colon cancer in two Scandinavian populations." *American Journal of Clinical Nutrition.* 31:S239–S242, 1978.

Mozaffarian, DS, Kumanyika, K, Lemaitre, RN, et al. "Cereal, fruit and vegetable fiber intake and the risk of cardiovascular disease in elderly individuals." *Journal of the American Medical Association.* 289(13):1659–1666, 2003.

Reinli, K, Block, G. "Phytoestrogen content of foods—a compendium of literature values." *Nutrition and Cancer.* 26:123–148, 1996.

Steffen, LM, Jacobs, DR, Jr, Murtaugh, MA, et al. "Whole grain intake is associated with lower body mass and greater insulin sensitivity among adolescents." *American Journal of Epidemiology.* 158(3):243–250, 2003.

Taylor, CG. "Chiro-inositol in buckwheat extract used to treat diabetic rats." *Journal of Agricultural and Food Chemistry.* December 2003.

Fruits

Hertog, MGL, Feskens, EGM, Hollman, PCH, et al. "Dietary antioxidant flavonoids and the risk of coronary heart disease: the Zutphen Elderly Study." *The Lancet.* 342:1007–1011, 1993.

Hertog, MGL, Hollman, PCH, Katan, MB. "Content of potentially anticarcinogenic flavonoids of 28 vegetables and 9 fruits commonly consumed in the Netherlands." *Journal of Agricultural and Food Chemistry.* 40:2379–2383, 1992.

Prior, R, et al. "Antioxidant capacity as influenced by total phenolic and anthocyanin content, maturity and variety of Vaccinium species." *Journal of Agricultural and Food Chemistry.* 46:2686–2693, 1998.

Spiller, GA, Moynihan, S, Butterfield, G. "Effects of sun-dried raisins on serum glucose: support for a convenient, plant-based snack food." *Vegetarian Nutrition: An International Journal.* 2(3):93–95, 1998.

Spiller, GA, Schultz, L, Spiller, M. "Sun-dried raisins help prevent oxidative DNA damage during intense athletic activity." *Journal of the American College of Nutrition.* 21(5):482, 2002.

Wang, H, Cao, G, Prior, R. "Total antioxidant capacity of fruits." *Journal of Agricultural Food Chemistry.* 44:701–705, 1996.

Vegetables, Fungi, and Seaweed

Agarwal, S, Rao, AV. "Tomato lycopene and its role in human health and chronic diseases." *Canadian Medical Association Journal.* 6:163, September 19, 2000.

Brown, JA, Fry, SC. "Novel O-D-galacturonoyl esters in the pectic polysaccharides of suspension cultured plant cells." *Plant Physiology.* 103(3):993–999, 1993.

Challier, B, Perarnau, JM, Viel, JF. "Garlic, onion and cereal fibre as protective factors for breast cancer: A French case control study." *European Journal of Epidemiology.* 14(8):737–747, 1998.

Chu, YF, Sun, J, Wu, X., et al. "Antioxidant and antiproliferative activities of common vegetables." *Journal of Agricultural and Food Chemistry.* 50:6910–6916, 2002.

Conaway, CC, Getahun, SM, Liebes, LL, et al. "Disposition of glucosinolates and sulforaphane in humans after ingestion of steamed and fresh broccoli." *Nutrition and Cancer.* 38(2):168–78, 2000.

Giovannucci, E, Rimm, EB, Stampfer, MJ, et al. "A prospective study of tomato products, lycopene, and prostate cancer risk." *Journal of the National Cancer Institute.* 94(5):391–98, 2002.

Grant, WB. "A multicountry ecologic study of risk and risk reduction factors for prostate cancer mortality." *European Urology.* 45:271–279, 2004.

Grube, BJ, Eng, ET, Kao, YC, et al. "White button mushroom phytochemicals inhibit aromatase activity and breast cancer cell proliferation." *Journal of Nutrition.* 131(12):3288–3293, 2001.

Hara, M, Hanaoka, T, Kobayishi, M, et al. "Cruciferous vegetables, mushrooms, and gastrointestinal cancer risks in multicenter, hospital-based, case-control study in Japan." *Nutrition and Cancer.* 46(2):138–47, 2003.

Hsing, AW, Chokkalingam, AP, Gao, YT, et al. "Allium vegetables and risk of prostate cancer: a population-based study." *Journal of the National Cancer Institute.* 94:1648–1651, 2002.

Ishii, T. "Feruloyl oligosaccharides from cell walls of suspension-cultured spinach cells and sugar beet pulp." *Plant Cell Physiology.* 35(4):701–704, 1994.

Lengsfeld, GC, Titgemeyer, F, Faller, G, et al. "Glycosylated compounds from okra inhibit adhesion of Helicobacter pylori to human gastric mucosa." *Journal of Agricultural and Food Chemistry.* 52(6):1495–1503, 2004.

Ng, ML, Yap, AT. "Inhibition of human colon carcinoma development by lentinan from shiitake mushrooms (Lentinus edodes)." *Journal of Alternative and Complementary Medicine.* 8(5):581–589, 2002.

Ninfali, P, Bacchiocca, M. "Polyphenols and antioxidant capacity of vegetables under fresh and frozen conditions." *Journal of Agricultural and Food Chemistry.* 51: 2222–2226, 2003.

Ruhe, RC, McDonald, RB. "Use of antioxidant nutrients in the prevention and treatment of type-2 diabetes." *Journal of the American College of Nutrition.* Oct 20(5 Suppl):363S–369S; discussion 381S–383S, 2001.

Sicilia, T, Niemeyer, HB, Honig, DM, et al. "Identification and stereochemical characterization of lignans in flaxseed and pumpkin seeds." *Journal of Agricultural and Food Chemistry.* 51:1181–1188, 2003.

Villasenor, IM, Domingo, AP. "Anticarcinogenicity potential of spinasterol isolated from squash flowers." *Teratogenesis Carcinogenesis and Mutagenesis.* 20(3):99–105, 2000.

Yamada, K, Yamada, Y, Fukuda, M, et al. "Bioavailability of dried asakusanori (Porphyra tenera) as a source of cobalamin (Vitamin B_{12})." *International Journal of Vitamin and Nutrition Research.* 69(6):412–418, 1999.

Zeisel, SH, Mar, MH, Howe, JC, et al. "Concentrations of choline-containing compounds and betaine in common foods." *Journal of Nutrition.* 133:1302–1307, May 2003.

Zhang, JT. "New drugs derived from medicinal plants." *Therapie.* 57(2):137–150, 2002.

Plant Extracts

Halvorsen, BL, Holte, K, Myhrstad, MCW, et al. "A systematic screening of total antioxidants in dietary plants." *Journal of Nutrition.* 132:461–471, 2002.

Kim, ND, Mehta, R, Yu, W, et al. "Chemopreventive and adjuvant therapeutic potential of pomegranate (*Punica granatum*) for human breast cancer." *Breast Cancer Research and Treatment.* 71:203–217, 2002.

Mori-Okamoto, JY, Otawara-Hamamoto, H, Yamato, H, et al. "Pomegranate extract improves a depressive state and bone properties in menopausal syndrome model ovariectomized mice." *Journal of Ethnopharmacology.* 92(1):93–101, May 2004.

Index

About the Authors

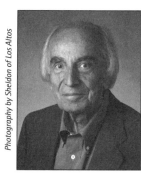

Dr. Gene Spiller has an M.S. and a Ph.D. in nutrition from the University of California, Berkeley, and is a Certified Nutrition Specialist (CNS), a fellow of the American College of Nutrition, and a member of other professional societies. His first scientific book on fiber was published in 1975 when fiber was beginning to find its proper place in nutrition. From 1982 to 2001, he edited three editions of the *CRC Handbook of Fiber in Human Nutrition*, and he has also authored books on nutrition for general audiences. He founded, and is director of the Sphera Foundation and the Health Research and Studies Center, both in Los Altos, California, and both involved in studying nutrition, writing books for scientific and lay audiences, and producing educational videos for schools.

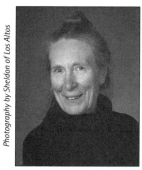

Monica Spiller first took a special interest in fiber in 1975 when she met Gene Spiller, at the time a newly published author of a book on dietary fiber. Born in London, she taught high school chemistry in England before coming to the San Francisco Bay area as an analytical chemist in pharmaceuticals. Since 1982, she has focused on ways to produce appealing wholegrain foods, in the process founding a company to promote the production of wholegrain bread and a non-profit organization, Whole Grain Connection, to further research and education. She has also been a contributing author to books and articles on whole grains and other healthy plant foods.